Cooking

FROM THE

Cupboard

Quick and Easy Low-Fat Meals

Jeanne Jones

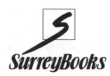

SurreyBooks

COOKING FROM THE CUPBOARD—Quick and Easy Low-Fat Meals
is published by Surrey Books, Inc., 230 E. Ohio St., Suite 120, Chicago, IL 60611.

First edition: 1 2 3 4 5

This book is manufactured in the United States of America.

Library of Congress Cataloging-in-Publication data:
Jones, Jeanne.
Cooking from the cupboard : Quick and easy low-fat meals / by Jeanne Jones.
   168p.   cm.
   Includes index.
   ISBN 0-940625-91-1 (pbk. : acid-free paper)
   1. Quick and easy cookery. 2. Low-fat diet—Recipes. I. Title.
TX833.5.J66 1995
641.5'63—dc20   95-13525
                                                CIP

Editorial and production: Bookcrafters, Inc., Chicago.
Design: Joan Sommers Design, Chicago.
Nutritional analyses: Linda R. Yoakam, M.S., R.D.

For free catalog and prices on quantity purchases, contact Surrey Books at the
address above.

This title is distributed to the trade by Publishers Group West.

CONTENTS

THIS BOOK IS truly a product of the times. It would not have been possible to write it even a few years ago because many of the healthier choices now available in pantry products simply did not exist.

Now, even canned soups are sporting labels touting their lower fat and sodium-reduced contents, and such notoriously high-fat products as mayonnaise and potato and corn chips are available fat free. Most dairy products, including many cheeses and ice creams, can be purchased non-fat as well as low fat. Water-packed tuna and chicken are outselling oil packed. Water- and juice-packed fruits are becoming more popular than their counterparts packed in heavy syrup. In other words, producers are really responding to consumer demands.

Also of enormous help in stocking a healthy pantry, are the new labeling laws. In 1994 it became mandatory to list both the ingredients and the nutritional information on all food products so that we really know what is inside the can, bottle, or box we are buying.

I still believe that the integrity of any dish depends on the quality of the ingredients used and that fresher is usually better. However, there are those times for all of us when everything seems to take longer than we had planned and we just can't get to the market. And natural disasters such as storms, floods, and earthquakes do occur. At these times we must rely totally on what we already have on hand, and a well-stocked pantry is not only a blessing but a real stress saver.

This is not meant to be an everyday cookbook. It is more a guidebook on how to use readily available, lighter pantry products to create delicious, satisfying, and healthy meals "in a hurry." This focus is on flavor and simplicity. The recipes are about convenience and economy rather than showmanship.

Nutritional information is provided for each recipe in this book based on software highly regarded by nutritionists and dietitians. However, this information is not infallible due to the many variables that affect nutritional data, such as: the exact sizes of fruits and vegetables, the error factor on the nutritional labels of canned and packaged foods, and variations in cooking techniques. Ingredients listed as "optional," "to taste," or as "garnish" are not included in the nutritional data. And when alternate choices of ingredients are given, the first-listed item is the one used to compute the nutritional data. In a word, the nutritional information should be used as a guideline for planning healthier meals, not as a basis for designing menus for people with strict dietary requirements.

To do the final testing on the recipes in this book, my husband and I packed all of the necessary pantry products and went out on a houseboat on Lake Mojave for ten days. Out on the lake, what we didn't have we couldn't get, making it an ideal testing site for this kind of menu planning. I am happy to report that we were both amazed and delighted by the quality and variety of ours meals.

When we returned home, I started serving some of my new pantry menus for dinner parties, purposely not telling my guests that they were dining on dishes prepared out of cans, bottles, and boxes. Not only did our guests rave about the food, but they almost always asked for the recipes!

Now, I urge *you* to stock your pantry, get out your can opener, and get rid of your stress—start "cooking from the cupboard."

PLANNING YOUR PANTRY

THE GOAL OF a well-stocked pantry should be to have enough food stored to prepare delicious and satisfying meals for at least two weeks.

Beyond bottled water, which is the most basic necessity, everyone's pantry planning will be different based on personal tastes and the amount of storage space available. And don't forget to include storerooms and the garage, as well as the kitchen, as possible storage areas.

In the kitchen we can now include our refrigerators and freezers, as well as our cupboards, as part of our total pantry system. However, if we lose electric power for any length of time, we also lose our cold storage. For this reason I place more emphasis on dry storage items, both for pantry planning and in most of the recipes in this book, than on ingredients requiring constant refrigeration. I would also urge you to keep cans of propane or Sterno on hand for heating your food if you live in an area where loss of power is a problem.

I am including a list of all the pantry items necessary to make the recipes in this book; use it as a guideline for stocking your own pantry. However, you certainly don't have to rush right out and buy everything on this list in order to have a well-stocked pantry. Start by buying the things you know you like and use most frequently while slowly adding to your herb and spice inventory.

Remember that this is only a guidebook to help you discover how to use pantry ingredients, not a blueprint that you must follow exactly. If you don't have the type of pasta, rice, or beans called for in a recipe, substitute another type. If you don't have canned chicken, use tuna, and vice versa. If you don't have the particular herb or spice called for, have fun experimenting with what you do have.

In restaurant kitchens they have a pantry control called "par" stock. Par is the number they never drop below. For example, if par on tomato sauce were one case, when only one case was left, another would be ordered. This is also a good system for running your home pantry. Let's say you frequently use canned, water-packed tuna and it would be frustrating to run out of it. You would make two cans your "par" on tuna, and when you only had two cans left, you would put tuna on your shopping list and buy two more cans.

If you have enough storage space, you can save a great deal of money buying the items you use most frequently at warehouse-type stores that offer huge discounts on cases. Also take advantage of weekend and seasonal specials to stock up on price-reduced staples. And don't forget to watch for sales on the non-food pantry supplies you need: cleaning products, foil, baggies, paper products, and the like.

There are a few obvious omissions in my dry pantry lists and they are not oversights. I have purposely not included dried parsley, cilantro, or lemon grass because I think they all taste more like dried alfalfa than their uniquely flavorful fresh counterparts. When a recipe calls for fresh parsley or cilantro and you don't have it, just omit it. If you don't have fresh lemon grass, substitute grated lemon rind to taste.

I have also omitted the dried Parmesan, Romano, and Cheddar cheeses that come in those round boxes because their fresh counterparts will last for months in the refrigerator and will keep for at least two weeks without refrigeration. Also, a little freshly grated Parmigiano-Reggiano, pecorino Romano, or high-quality aged Cheddar can make a simple pantry dish seem truly gourmet, while a bit of the boxed stuff can ruin the taste of an otherwise excellent, totally fresh culinary creation.

The reason I have omitted bouillon cubes of all types is because I don't like their taste. I think that canned stocks, broths, and consommés are a much more viable alternative for the "real" thing.

Dry Pantry Basics

Flour
    Whole wheat   Unbleached all-purpose

Sugar
    White   Dark brown
    Light brown

Dry, non-fat powdered instant milk	Cornstarch
"Just Whites"	Gelatin, unflavored
Cocoa	Light biscuit and pancake mix
Coffee	Graham cracker crumbs
Instant coffee	Graham cracker pie crust, baked
Tea	and packaged
Salt	Potato Buds
Baking powder	Cornbread mix
Baking soda	

Cereals and Grains
  Cornmeal
  Corn grits
  Oatmeal
  Quinoa

  Rye berries
  Bulgar (cracked wheat)
  Millet
  Wheat bran
  Mixed grain kashi

Dry Cereals
  All Bran
  Shredded Wheat
  Non-fat granola

  Puffed rice, wheat, corn, and Kashi
  Grape-Nuts

Dry Pasta
  Spaghetti
  Shells
  Linguini
  Bow ties

  Couscous
  Rigatoni
  Rotelli
  etc.

Rice
  White
  Instant white
  Jasmine

  Quick-cooking brown
  Quick-cooking wild
  Arborio

Beans
  Black
  Pinto
  Kidney
  Garbanzo
  Small white

  Cannellini
  Lentils
  Black-eyed peas
  Split peas

Shelf-stable tofu*

Imitation bacon chips

Dried Fruit*
  Raisins
  Prunes
  Apricots

  Apples, unsulfured
  Dates
  Figs

Dried Vegetables
  Dried tomatoes

  Mushrooms

*Should be refrigerated when opened

Fresh Vegetables
    Onions   Potatoes
    Garlic

Herbs and Spices

Herbs and spices are extremely important in healthy cooking. They contain practically no calories and, when used liberally, they can compensate for salt. Also, there are a number of good herb and spice blends now on the market that are completely salt free and excellent for seasoning dishes of all types.

Herbs and spices give every dish its individual personality. You can change the whole character of a recipe simply by using different seasonings. For example, you can take a basic chicken recipe and change the flavor to Italian by adding oregano, to Indian by adding curry powder, to French with a little thyme or tarragon, to Scandinavian with dill, to Asian by adding ginger, or to Southwestern with cumin and chili powder.

When using dried herbs and spices that are not powdered, it is essential to crush them using a mortar and pestle to release their full aroma. When you start using more herbs and spices in your cooking, you will be amazed at how much better everything will taste and how much your reputation as a creative cook will be enhanced.

Store your herbs and spices in a cool place where they are not exposed to sunlight, and alphabetize them for easy access. Alphabetizing them may not seem important to you now, but as you acquire more herbs and spices it will save you both time and frustration.

Allspice, whole and ground	Dill seeds
Anise, seeds and ground	Dill weed
Bay leaves	Fennel, seeds and ground
Basil	Garlic powder and flakes
Black peppercorns	Ginger, ground
Cayenne	Juniper berries
Cardamom, ground	Mace
Caraway seeds	Marjoram
Celery, seeds and ground	Mustard, seeds and powdered
Cinnamon, sticks and ground	Nutmeg, whole and ground
Chili powder	Onion flakes
Cloves, whole and ground	Oregano
Cumin, seeds and ground	Paprika
Curry powder	Poppy seeds
Coriander, ground	Red pepper flakes

Rosemary	Tarragon
Saffron	Thyme
Sage	Turmeric
Sesame seeds	White pepper

Blends

Cajun	Southwestern
Italian	Thai

Bottles and Jars

Water, sparkling and still

Extracts

Almond	Vanilla
Coconut	Vanilla Butter and Nut
Rum	

Condiments, Seasonings, Sauces, and Salad Dressings

Low-fat and fat-free salad dressings*	Pickle relish*
Mayonnaise, low-fat and fat-free*	Angostura bitters
Mustard, Dijon and brown*	Liquid smoke
Horseradish*	Sodium-reduced soy sauce
Salsa*	Sodium-reduced teriyaki sauce
Pesto sauce*	Thai fish sauce
Pasta and pizza sauces*	Worcestershire sauce*
Barbecue sauce*	Tabasco
Chili sauce*	Capers*
Catsup*	Olives*
Hoisin*	Pimientos*
Pickles*	Roasted red peppers*

Clam Juice*

Vinegars

White	Balsamic
Cider	Raspberry
Rice	Sherry
Red wine	

*Should be refrigerated when opened

Oils
    Canola   Dark sesame
    Olive, extra-virgin   Walnut

Syrups, Jams, and Jellies
    Honey   All-fruit jams and jellies*
    Maple syrup   Pepper jelly*
    Corn syrup

Peanut butter (unhomogenized, or
    old fashioned)*

Wines
    Sherry   Red, dry
    Port   Vermouth
    White, dry   Madeira

Liquors and Liqueurs
    Brandy   Pernod
    Rum   Sake
    Amaretto   Mirin (sweet sake)
    Grand Marnier or any orange
       liqueur

Canned Goods*

Nuts (also available in bags and bulk)*
    Almonds   Pine nuts
    Peanuts   Walnuts
    Pecans

Soup Stock (Store other than fat-free chicken
    and beef stock in the refrigerator so that the
    fat will congeal on top and be removed
    easily before using.)
    Sodium-reduced chicken   Vegetable
    Sodium-reduced beef

*All canned goods should be refrigerated when opened

Soups

Cream of mushroom, fat- and sodium-reduced

Cream of chicken

Cream of celery

Tomato, sodium-reduced

Pea

Potato

Onion

Vegetarian chili

Milk, evaporated, skim

Juices

Apple

Pineapple

Tomato

V-8

Fruits

Peaches, sliced, in water

Pineapple, crushed and chunks, in juice

Pears, in juice

Mandarin oranges, in juice

Lychees, in syrup

Vegetables

Artichoke hearts, in water

Hearts of palm, in water

Water chestnuts, in water

Green beans

Peas

Corn

Creamed corn

Carrots

Potatoes and new potatoes

Pumpkin, solid pack

Mushrooms

Bamboo shoots

Green chilies, diced and whole

Onions

Tomatoes, whole, chopped, seasoned, sauce, and paste

Caponata

Beans

Black

Cannellini

Garbanzo (chickpeas)

Kidney

Pinto

Fat-free refried

Vegetarian refried

Seafood

Clams, chopped and minced

Clam juice

Crab, white

Lobster

Oysters

Tuna, in water

Salmon

Shrimp

*All canned goods should be refrigerated when opened

Poultry
    Chicken, chunk style in water   Turkey, in water

Meat
    Beef, roast, in gravy   Ham, chunk
    Corned beef

Refrigerator Basics

This list includes only items that should always be stored in the refrigerator, opened or not. Among dry pantry items, those that should be refrigerated after they are opened have an asterisk (*) after them.

Milk, non-fat, low-fat, and buttermilk
Yogurt, non-fat and low-fat
Fresh, aged cheeses
Fresh tofu
Eggs
Liquid egg substitutes
Butter and margarine
Sour cream, fat-free and light
Refrigerator bread dough, such as pizza and biscuit
Bread
Apples
Citrus fruits
Cabbage and coleslaw mixes
Parsley
Cilantro
Lemon grass (if you don't use it often, keep it in the freezer)

Freezer Basics

Meat
    Lean ground beef   Lean, cubed stew meat

Ice cream, light (low-fat ice milk or fat-free)
Frozen yogurt, non-fat or low-fat
Whipped toppings, light
Phyllo pastry
Bread dough
Leftovers

Vegetables
    Chopped onions   Spinach, chopped and leaf
    Peas   Stir-fry and stew mixes
    Corn   Any others you like and use often
    Broccoli

Fruit, unsweetened
   Blueberries   Peaches, sliced
   Cherries, pitted   Raspberries
   Cranberries   Strawberries

Juice concentrates
   Apple   etc.
   Orange

Seafood
   Crab   Shrimp

Poultry
   Chicken breasts, skinned and   Turkey, ground
      boned

Shopping Tips

The grocery industry is doing everything possible to make shopping in the nineties more fun. In many suburban areas the supermarket is becoming the social gathering place of choice for many people who meet after work for coffee or a glass of wine and do their shopping together. No matter how large or small your favorite market may be, there are some things you can do to make shopping easier.

Keep a shopping list in your kitchen, and every time you run out of something, or are down to "par," put it on the list. Before going to the market, plan your weekly menu and add all of the necessary ingredients to your list. Never go to the market without a list. Just having a list can save you lots of money because it will keep you from falling into the trap of impulse buying, or "eye-level shopping."

One-stop shopping is not always possible. You may have to go to a health food store for some of the items on your list such as unsulfured dried apples and some of the whole-grain products. Ethnic markets might be the best source for others, like arborio rice, Thai fish sauce, and lemon grass.

Read the labels! Now that we have mandatory labeling on most food items, you can really be sure of what is inside the can, bottle, or box. Pay close attention to the nutritional information given, and be sure to read how many servings are in the container. Sometimes the calories and fat seem low—until you realize that the information given is for each serving and there are four servings in the container.

To help you estimate the percentage of fat in any item, multiply the grams of fat by ten. Even though the actual number of calories for each gram of fat is nine, it's a whole lot faster, and easier, to round off to ten. Your daily eating goal should be no more than 30 percent of calories from fat.

Try to avoid preservatives. They are usually long, chemical-sounding names in the ingredients list. A good rule of thumb is, if there are too many ingredients listed that you can't pronounce, don't buy the product.

THESE RECIPES ARE designed for quick, easy, and economical meals. When possible, I have used only one cooking method in each recipe. Rather than starting something on top of the stove and then transferring it to the oven, most dishes are started and finished in one place and in the same pot or pan. This saves both time and energy *and* it makes clean up easier!

I also routinely use up the entire amount in the cans called for in all of the recipes in this book. I never ask you to use only a part of the contents and then figure out what you are going to do with the rest of it. For example, when a recipe calls for canned evaporated milk, it always uses the entire 12 ounces (1½ cups) in the can.

If a recipe calls for fresh non-fat milk and you don't have any in the refrigerator, just make the amount you need for the recipe using dry non-fat milk powder and water. You can also buy dry powdered buttermilk to avoid buying a whole quart of the fresh if you only need a cup of buttermilk in a recipe.

If you have fresh herbs and prefer to use them instead of the dried herbs called for in a recipe, a good rule of thumb is to use three times as much. The only exception is rosemary, because the flavor of the fresh herb is just as intense as the dried; so use the same amount.

Dried beans and peas are more economical than canned, but they take much longer to prepare and therefore are not as convenient. For this reason I have used canned beans in all of the recipes in this book. In fact, I have had readers tell me that when the first thing they read in a recipe is "soak the beans overnight," they routinely turn the page to see if they can find a recipe that can be made and put on the table in thirty minutes instead of tomorrow. If you are cooking for a large family and don't want to spend the extra money for canned beans, here is a time-saving tip when using dried beans and peas. Soak lots of beans overnight and store them in zip lock bags in the freezer. Then when you want to use them in a recipe, even though they still have to be cooked for an hour, at least they're ready to put on the stove.

Almost all of these pantry recipes can be adapted to what is now called "speed scratch" or "assembly" cooking simply by replacing some of the pantry products with fresh ingredients. Buy fresh fruits and vegetables at the salad bar section in your supermarket, already cut up and ready to use. This not only saves preparation time but allows you to buy, albeit at a higher price, just the amounts you need of each item.

Fresh or frozen seafood, poultry, and meat can also be used instead of the canned products called for in strictly pantry recipes. In fact, when possible, I would encourage you to make these substitutions, particularly in the poultry and meat categories. Canned seafood is, for the most part, a higher-quality product. The only two categories of canned seafood I don't recommend are shrimp and oysters. Instead, keep shrimp in the freezer and buy jars of fresh, shucked oysters when you want them for oyster stew. Shrimp and oysters can be replaced in recipes with canned tuna, crab, or clams.

The highest quality canned poultry product is chunk white chicken packed in water. It is also the most expensive. Therefore, unless you are limited to canned ingredients, I recommend keeping chicken breasts in the freezer.

The only way you can buy canned beef is to get roast beef in gravy from either Brazil or Argentina, and I don't happen to like the way it tastes. That is why I always rinse, drain, and shred it in my recipes. Also, I always call for canned chunk ham in the five-ounce cans rather than the larger canned hams; it's ready to use and you don't have any leftovers. If you prefer to buy the larger canned hams, just chop three-quarters of a cup of it for each can called for in a recipe.

Pantry recipes tend to be higher in sodium content. If you want to lower the sodium content of any of these recipes, you can find reduced-sodium products in the health food section of most supermarkets and in all health food stores. However, you can usually stay within the American Heart Association's guidelines for daily sodium intake simply by mixing and matching the recipes in this book.

ONE

Sauces

AND

Dressings

There is now an abundance of both low-fat and fat-free sauces and salad dressings available in all supermarkets. However, because it is so easy to make some of the basic sauces and dressings from scratch, and so much less expensive, I am including some of my favorite recipes in this chapter.

Apple Butter 🌀 Barbecue Sauce 🌀 Dill Sauce

Horseradish Sauce 🌀 Light Aioli

Oil-Free Salad Dressing 🌀 Salsa

Apple Butter

There are many good brands of sugar-free apple butter available, but I still prefer making my own. It is tastier, less expensive, and it will keep for weeks in the refrigerator. You usually have to go to a health food store to find unsulfured dried apples, but it is well worth the trip because they are so much more flavorful than the lighter-colored, sulfured variety—and they make a much better quality apple butter.

¼ lb. (2 cups) dried, unsulfured, sliced apples
1 teaspoon ground cinnamon
½ teaspoon ground allspice
⅛ teaspoon ground cloves
2 cups unsweetened apple juice

1. Combine all ingredients in a large saucepan and bring to a boil over medium heat. Reduce heat to low and simmer, covered, 20 minutes, stirring occasionally.

2. Remove from heat, spoon into a blender or food processor, and blend until smooth. Cool to room temperature. Spoon mixture into a container with a tight-fitting lid and store in refrigerator. (Makes 2 cups.)

SERVES 32 (1-tablespoon servings)

Per Serving:	*Exchanges:*
Calories: 21	Milk: 0.0
% Calories from Fat: 2	Vegetable: 0.0
Fat (gm): 0	Fruit: 0.5
Saturated Fat (gm): 0	Bread: 0.0
Cholesterol (mg): 0	Meat: 0.0
Sodium (mg): 5.2	Fat: 0.0
Protein (gm): 0.1	
Carbohydrate (gm): 5.5	

Barbecue Sauce

1 medium onion, finely chopped, *or* 1½ cups frozen chopped onions

2 tablespoons water

½ cup tomato catsup

½ teaspoon grated lemon rind

2 tablespoons freshly squeezed lemon juice

1½ tablespoons Worcestershire sauce

1 tablespoon cider vinegar

¾ teaspoon dry mustard

6 tablespoons frozen unsweetened apple juice concentrate

¼ teaspoon Liquid Smoke

1. Combine onions and water in a small saucepan, and cook about 10 minutes until onions are soft and translucent. Add all other ingredients except Liquid Smoke. Mix well and bring to a boil. Reduce heat to medium and cook, uncovered, until thick, about 30 minutes.

2. Remove from heat, add Liquid Smoke, and mix well. Pour into a blender container and blend until smooth. Cool to room temperature, then refrigerate in a tightly covered container. (Makes 1½ cups.)

SERVES 6 (¼-cup servings)

Per Serving:	*Exchanges:*
Calories: 67	Milk: 0.0
% Calories from Fat: 4	Vegetable: 0.0
Fat (gm): 0.3	Fruit: 1.0
Saturated Fat (gm): 0	Bread: 0.0
Cholesterol (mg): 0	Meat: 0.0
Sodium (mg): 312	Fat: 0.0
Protein (gm): 0.9	
Carbohydrate (gm): 16.5	

Dill Sauce

This sauce is wonderful on seafood of all types. I always serve it with the Salmon Mousse on page 94. When possible, make it a day before you plan to serve it so the flavors can "marry."

1 cup fat-free sour cream

½ cup fat-free mayonnaise

½ teaspoon salt

1 teaspoon dried tarragon, crushed

1½ teaspoons dried dill weed, crushed

1. Combine all ingredients in a bowl and mix well. Cover and refrigerate. (Makes 1½ cups.)

SERVES 24 (1-tablespoon servings)

Per Serving:	*Exchanges:*
Calories: 10	Milk: 0.0
% Calories from Fat: 1	Vegetable: 0.0
Fat (gm): 0	Fruit: 0.0
Saturated Fat (gm): 0	Bread: 0.0
Cholesterol (mg): 0	Meat: 0.0
Sodium (mg): 114	Fat: 0.0
Protein (gm): 0.7	
Carbohydrate (gm): 2	

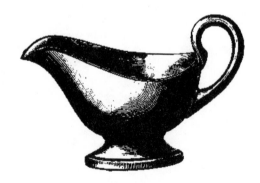

Horseradish Sauce

This sauce should be made ahead of time to give the flavors a chance to "marry." However, if you want to use it immediately, it is still a very tasty topping for vegetables, seafood, poultry, and meat of all types. You can create your own variations to this basic recipe by adding one or a combination of your favorite herbs.

¼ cup prepared horseradish

½ cup fat-free mayonnaise

½ cup fat-free sour cream

½ teaspoon Dijon mustard

1 teaspoon lemon juice

¼ teaspoon salt

⅛ teaspoon freshly ground black pepper

1. Combine all ingredients in a bowl and mix well. Cover and refrigerate overnight, when possible, before using. (Makes 1 cup.)

SERVES 16 (1-tablespoon servings)

Per Serving:	*Exchanges:*
Calories: 12	Milk: 0.0
% Calories from Fat: 1	Vegetable: 0.0
Fat (gm): 0	Fruit: 0.0
Saturated Fat (gm): 0	Bread: 0.0
Cholesterol (mg): 0	Meat: 0.0
Sodium (mg): 176	Fat: 0.0
Protein (gm): 0.5	
Carbohydrate (gm): 2.6	

Light Aioli

Aioli is a French garlic-mayonnaise from the region of Provence. It is classically made with egg yolks, crushed garlic, olive oil, salt, and sometimes a little lemon juice. In this recipe I have used tofu as the base and just enough good extra-virgin olive oil to add flavor and smooth out the texture. Although the percentage of fat is still high, it is not meant to be eaten by itself but as a condiment with other foods. I am delighted with my cholesterol-free, lower-calorie aioli, and I hope you will be too.

1 10½-ounce package silken firm tofu

2 tablespoons lemon juice

2 tablespoons extra-virgin olive oil

3 garlic cloves, halved

½ teaspoon salt

⅛ teaspoon freshly ground black pepper

1. Combine all ingredients in a blender or food processor, and blend until satin smooth. Store tightly covered in refrigerator. (Makes 1¼ cups.)

SERVES 10 (2-tablespoon servings)

Per Serving:	*Exchanges:*
Calories: 44	Milk: 0.0
% Calories from Fat: 70	Vegetable: 0.0
Fat (gm): 3.5	Fruit: 0.0
Saturated Fat (gm): 0.5	Bread: 0.5
Cholesterol (mg): 0	Meat: 0.0
Sodium (mg): 117	Fat: 0.5
Protein (gm): 2.1	
Carbohydrate (gm): 1.4	

Oil-Free Salad Dressing

½ cup red wine vinegar

¼ teaspoon freshly ground black pepper

½ teaspoon salt

1 tablespoon sugar

2 garlic cloves, finely chopped (2 teaspoons)

2 teaspoons Worcestershire sauce

1 tablespoon Dijon-style mustard

2 tablespoons freshly squeezed lemon juice

1 cup water

1. Combine all ingredients and mix well. Refrigerate in a container with a tight-fitting lid. Dressing will keep for months. (Makes 2 cups.)

SERVES 16 (2-tablespoon servings)

Per Serving:	*Exchanges:*
Calories: 8	Milk: 0.0
% Calories from Fat: 9	Vegetable: 0.0
Fat (gm): 0.1	Fruit: 0.0
Saturated Fat (gm): 0	Bread: 0.0
Cholesterol (mg): 0	Meat: 0.0
Sodium (mg): 85	Fat: 0.0
Protein (gm): 0.1	
Carbohydrate (gm): 1.6	

Variations (nutritional data will be altered)

Italian: Add 1 teaspoon each crushed dried tarragon, oregano, and basil.

Cumin: Add ½ teaspoon ground cumin.

Curry: Add 1 teaspoon curry powder.

Tarragon: Add 1 tablespoon crushed dried tarragon.

Creamy Salad Dressing: Add ¼ cup non-fat plain yogurt, *or* non-fat sour cream.

Sun-Dried Tomato Vinaigrette: Bring ½ cup of water called for in recipe to a boil and pour over ¼ cup dry sun-dried tomatoes. Allow to stand 10 minutes, then process in a blender along with remaining ½ cup water. Pour mixture into dressing.

Salsa

There is a variety of really good, already prepared salsas available in all super-markets. You can choose among fresh and bottled, red and green, mild, medium, and really hot. However, if you need salsa immediately, here is an easy-to-make recipe, using only standard pantry ingredients.

1 14½-ounce can chopped tomatoes, drained

1 4-ounce can diced green chilies

½ medium onion, chopped, *or* ¾ cup frozen chopped onions

1 garlic clove, pressed or minced

¾ teaspoon ground oregano, crushed

¾ teaspoon ground cumin

¼ teaspoon freshly ground black pepper

1 tablespoon lemon, *or* lime, juice

3 tablespoons chopped fresh cilantro (optional)

1. Combine all ingredients in a bowl and mix well. (Makes 2 cups.)

SERVES 8 (¼-cup servings)

Per Serving:	*Exchanges:*
Calories: 21	Milk: 0.0
% Calories from Fat: 8	Vegetable: 1.0
Fat (gm): 0.2	Fruit: 0.0
Saturated Fat (gm): 0	Bread: 0.0
Cholesterol (mg): 0	Meat: 0.0
Sodium (mg): 88	Fat: 0.0
Protein (gm): 0.8	
Carbohydrate (gm): 4.7	

TWO

Soups

This chapter offers a wide variety of soups, often using more than one canned soup as basic ingredients. Many of these soups are actually one-dish meals while others can double as sauces for other dishes.

Gazpacho ⊚ Cold Spiced Peach Soup ⊚ Pear and Roquefort Cheese Soup ⊚ Curried Pumpkin Soup Curried Chicken Bisque ⊚ Sherried Pea Soup Peanut Soup ⊚ Black Bean Soup ⊚ Minestrone Spinach Soup ⊚ Cheddar Cheese Soup ⊚ Crab Bisque Oyster Stew ⊚ Clam Chowder ⊚ Seafood Soup ⊚ Senegalese Soup ⊚ Southwestern Corn and Chicken Soup ⊚ Thai Chicken and Water Chestnut Soup ⊚ Turkey and Rice Soup

Gazpacho

This cold Mexican soup is even better if made the day before you plan to serve it, and it will keep for several days in the refrigerator. It can also be served as a salsa, or sauce, on salads or any Southwestern dish.

1 medium onion, chopped, *or* 1½ cups frozen chopped onions

1 garlic clove, pressed or minced

1 7-ounce jar roasted red sweet peppers, drained, chopped

1 14½-ounce can chopped tomatoes, undrained

2 11½-ounce cans V-8 juice

¼ teaspoon freshly ground black pepper

⅛ teaspoon ground cumin

½ teaspoon Worcestershire sauce

3 tablesoons lemon juice

¼ teaspoon Tabasco sauce, *or* to taste

1. Combine all ingredients and mix well. Refrigerate until cold before serving. (Makes 6 cups.)

SERVES 8 (¾-cup servings)

Per Serving:	*Exchanges:*
Calories: 42	Milk: 0.0
% Calories from Fat: 4	Vegetable: 1.5
Fat (gm): 0.2	Fruit: 0.0
Saturated Fat (gm): 0	Bread: 0.0
Cholesterol (mg): 0	Meat: 0.0
Sodium (mg): 356	Fat: 0.0
Protein (gm): 1.4	
Carbohydrate (gm): 9.6	

Cold Spiced Peach Soup

This refreshing, cold soup can either be served as an appetizer or a dessert.

1 16-ounce can sliced peaches, packed in water, no sugar added, undrained

2 teaspoons sugar

½ teaspoon ground cinnamon

¼ teaspoon ground allspice

Dash ground clove

½ teaspoon vanilla extract

¼ cup non-fat plain yogurt

1. Combine all ingredients in a blender or food processor and puree. Chill well before serving. (Makes 2 cups.)

SERVES 4 (½-cup servings)

Per Serving:	*Exchanges:*
Calories: 46	Milk: 0.0
% Calories from Fat: 2	Vegetable: 0.0
Fat (gm): 0.1	Fruit: 1.0
Saturated Fat (gm): 0	Bread: 0.0
Cholesterol (mg): 0.3	Meat: 0.0
Sodium (mg): 14	Fat: 0.0
Protein (gm): 1.3	
Carbohydrate (gm): 10.6	

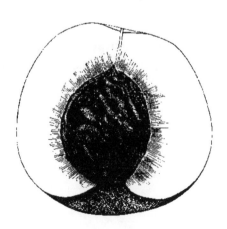

Pear and Roquefort Cheese Soup

The secret of the flavor in this unusual and delicious soup is the distinctive taste of Roquefort combined with the sweetness of pears. Unlike many other blue-veined cheeses, Roquefort is made only from sheep's milk and produced only in the Caves of Roquefort in France. Both Monterey Jack and cottage cheese are added for texture. If you have any soup leftover, serve it cold as a salad dressing, or warm it up and use it as a sauce on poached or grilled chicken.

- 1 medium onion, chopped, or 1½ cups frozen chopped onions
- 1 16-ounce can peeled Bartlett pears in lightly sweetened juice, undrained
- 1 14½-ounce can fat-free, sodium-reduced chicken stock
- 2 ounces fat-reduced Monterey Jack cheese, grated (½ cup)
- 2 ounces Roquefort cheese, crumbled (½ cup)
- ½ cup non-fat cottage cheese

1. Cook onion in a heavy pot, covered, over medium-low heat about 10 minutes or until soft and translucent, adding a little water if necessary to prevent scorching.

2. Drain pears and add pear juice to onions in the pot. Dice pears and set aside.

3. Add chicken stock to pot and bring to a boil. Simmer, uncovered, over medium heat until reduced by ⅓, about 10 minutes. Remove from heat and puree in a blender or food processor. Pour puree back into pot through a strainer, pressing all liquid through with back of a spoon.

4. Add grated Jack cheese and place pot back over heat until melted. Do not allow to boil.

5. Remove from heat and stir in diced pears, Roquefort, and cottage cheese. Soup can be served at room temperature or covered and refrigerated until cold. (Make 4 cups.)

SERVES 8 (½-cup servings)

Per Serving:	*Exchanges:*
Calories: 95	Milk: 0.0
% Calories from Fat: 32	Vegetable: 0.0
Fat (gm): 3.5	Fruit: 0.5
Saturated Fat (gm): 2.1	Bread: 0.0
Cholesterol (mg): 12.2	Meat: 1.0
Sodium (mg): 300	Fat: 0.0
Protein (gm): 7.1	
Carbohydrate (gm): 9.4	

Curried Pumpkin Soup

The giant orange spheres we see growing in roadside fields, all looking like they're vying to become Cinderella's coach for the ball or destined to be carved into Jack-O-Lanterns for Halloween, are not the best pumpkins for eating. Their flesh is watery, stringy, and lacking in flavor. The best variety for cooking, often called sugar pumpkins, are much smaller in size and have a sweeter flavor and finer-textured flesh. These tastier varieties are still time consuming to prepare. Canned solid-pack pumpkin is an excellent substitute, and it is available all year around. Although pumpkins make delicious pies, they are a standard vegetable in many other parts of the world. This spicy and unusual curried pumpkin soup is based on one of my favorite African recipes. It can be served hot or cold, but I like it best just a little warmer than room temperature.

1 medium onion, chopped, *or* 1½ cups chopped frozen onions

1 cup unsweetened applesauce

1 tablespoon dark brown sugar

1 teaspoon curry powder

1 teaspoon ground cumin

½ teaspoon ground ginger

¼ teaspoon ground cardamom

½ teaspoon salt

¼ teaspoon freshly ground black pepper

1 16-ounce can solid-pack pumpkin

1 14½-ounce can fat-free, sodium-reduced chicken stock

1 12-ounce can evaporated skim milk

1. Cook onion in a heavy pot or soup kettle, covered, over medium-low heat about 10 minutes or until soft and translucent, adding a little water if necessary to prevent scorching.

2. Add applesauce, brown sugar, curry, cumin, ginger, cardamom, salt, and pepper and cook over medium heat, stirring frequently, 5 more minutes. Add pumpkin and chicken stock and bring to a boil. Reduce heat to low and cook, covered, 20 minutes.

3. Remove from heat and add milk. Pour mixture into a blender or food processor, in 2 batches, and puree. Serve as is or pour through a strainer for a smoother-textured soup. (Makes 6 cups.)

SERVES 8 (¾-cup servings)

Per Serving:
Calories: 86
% Calories from Fat: 4
Fat (gm): 0.4
Saturated Fat (gm): 0.1
Cholesterol (mg): 1.3
Sodium (mg): 264
Protein (gm): 5.2
Carbohydrate (gm): 16.5

Exchanges:
Milk: 0.5
Vegetable: 0.0
Fruit: 0.0
Bread: 0.5
Meat: 0.0
Fat: 0.0

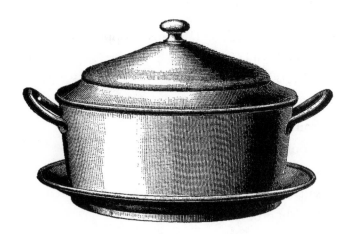

Curried Chicken Bisque

This delicious, mildly flavored curry soup can double as an entree served over cooked rice or pasta. It is also good cold. When serving it cold, I puree the soup in a blender with 3 tablespoons of mango chutney and serve it with cinnamon rice cakes.

1 10¾-ounce can fat-reduced cream of chicken soup

1 10¾-ounce can fat-reduced cream of mushroom soup

1 12-ounce can evaporated skim milk

1 teaspoon curry powder

½ teaspoon turmeric

¼ teaspoon ground ginger

1 10-ounce can chunk white chicken, in water

1. Combine chicken and mushroom soups in a blender and puree.

2. Combine the pureed soups with all remaining ingredients, except chicken, in a saucepan and slowly bring to a simmer. Add chicken, mix well, and serve. If making ahead of time, reheat to desired temperature but do not boil. (Makes 4 cups.)

SERVES 4 (1-cup servings)

Per Serving:	*Exchanges:*
Calories: 227	Milk: 0.5
% Calories from Fat: 30	Vegetable: 0.0
Fat (gm): 7.2	Fruit: 0.0
Saturated Fat (gm): 1.7	Bread: 1.0
Cholesterol (mg): 45	Meat: 2.0
Sodium (mg): 764	Fat: 0.0
Protein (gm): 22.6	
Carbohydrate (gm): 16.2	

Sherried Pea Soup

This is a quick and easy soup that is equally good served hot or cold. For a creamier soup, you can substitute one twelve-ounce can evaporated skim milk for the chicken stock called for in this recipe.

1 10¾-ounce can condensed green pea soup

1 14½-ounce can fat-free, sodium-reduced chicken stock

2 tablespoons sherry, *or* to taste

Lemon zest for garnish (optional)

1. Combine pea soup and chicken stock in a saucepan and slowly bring to a boil over medium-low heat. Add sherry and serve hot, or cool to room temperature and refrigerate until cold. Top each serving with a pinch of lemon zest, if desired. (Makes 3 cups.)

SERVES 4 (¾-cup servings)

Per Serving:
Calories: 113
% Calories from Fat: 13
Fat (gm): 1.7
Saturated Fat (gm): 0.8
Cholesterol (mg): 0
Sodium (mg): 686
Protein (gm): 6.6
Carbohydrate (gm): 16.3

Exchanges:
Milk: 0.0
Vegetable: 2.0
Fruit: 0.0
Bread: 0.5
Meat: 0.0
Fat: 0.0

Peanut Soup

This soup really needs the one-fourth cup of peanut butter called for in order to have the rich peanut flavor that makes it so delicious. For this reason, more than 30 percent of the calories come from fat. To balance your meal, I suggest serving it with vegetables and a whole-grain roll.

2 teaspoons canola oil

1 small onion, finely chopped, *or* 1 cup frozen chopped onions

2½ tablespoons all-purpose flour

1 teaspoon curry powder

¼ teaspoon salt

1 14½-ounce can fat-free, sodium-reduced chicken stock, boiling

¼ cup unhomogenized (old fashioned) smooth peanut butter

1 12-ounce can evaporated skim milk

1. Heat oil in a saucepan over medium-low heat. Add onion and cook, stirring frequently, until translucent. Add flour, curry powder, and salt and cook, stirring constantly, 3 minutes.

2. Pour in boiling chicken stock and whisk until smooth. Add peanut butter and cook until melted and slightly thickened. Slowly add milk and heat to serving temperature. Do not allow to boil. (Makes 4 cups.)

SERVES 8 (½-cup servings)

Per Serving:	*Exchanges:*
Calories: 113	Milk: 0.5
% Calories from Fat: 41	Vegetable: 0.0
Fat (gm): 5.4	Fruit: 0.0
Saturated Fat (gm): 1	Bread: 0.0
Cholesterol (mg): 1.3	Meat: 0.5
Sodium (mg): 230	Fat: 1.0
Protein (gm): 6.9	
Carbohydrate (gm): 10.2	

Black Bean Soup

The Cubans claim to have created this robust soup, and they serve it over rice as a main dish. It is also excellent served as a first course, with a dollop of light sour cream and chopped green onions.

½ medium onion, chopped, *or* ¾ cup frozen chopped onions

1 garlic clove, pressed or minced

1 4-ounce can diced green chilies

2 15-ounce cans black beans, undrained

1 14½-ounce can fat-free, sodium-reduced chicken stock

1 teaspoon ground cumin

¼ teaspoon freshly ground black pepper

1 tablespoon red wine vinegar

¼ cup sherry

1. Combine onion, garlic, and green chilies in a saucepan and cook, covered, over low heat 10 minutes or until onion is translucent.

2. Put 1 can of black beans in a blender. Add can of chicken stock and puree. Pour pureed beans into cooked onion mixture. Stir in remaining can of beans and all other ingredients, except sherry, and bring to a boil. Reduce heat to low and simmer 15 minutes. Add sherry and simmer 5 more minutes. (Makes 6 cups.)

SERVES 8 (¾-cup servings)

Per Serving:
Calories: 108
% Calories from Fat: 7
Fat (gm): 1
Saturated Fat (gm): 0
Cholesterol (mg): 0
Sodium (mg): 413
Protein (gm): 9.9
Carbohydrate (gm): 20.6

Exchanges:
Milk: 0.0
Vegetable: 0.0
Fruit: 0.0
Bread: 1.5
Meat: 0.0
Fat: 0.0

Minestrone

This hearty Italian soup makes a wonderful vegetarian entree served either with crusty bread or Fast Focaccia (Pizza Bread) on page 130.

1 medium onion, chopped, *or* 1½ cups frozen chopped onions

2 garlic cloves, pressed or minced

1 14½-ounce can fat-free, sodium-reduced chicken, *or* vegetable stock

¼ cup dry white wine

¼ teaspoon freshly ground black pepper

¾ teaspoon dried rosemary, crushed

1 teaspoon chili powder

1 14½-ounce can chopped tomatoes, undrained

1 15-ounce can dark red kidney beans, undrained

1 8-ounce can Italian green beans, drained

1 cup shredded cabbage, *or* coleslaw mix

½ cup dry spaghetti (2 ounces), broken into 1-inch pieces

½ cup shredded Parmesan cheese

1. Combine onion and garlic and cook, covered, over low heat 10 minutes or until onion is translucent, adding a little water if necessary to prevent scorching.

2. Add all remaining ingredients, except spaghetti and cheese, and bring to a boil. Add spaghetti and cook 12 minutes. Add cheese and stir until cheese is melted. (Makes 7 cups.)

SERVES 7 (1-cup servings)

Per Serving:	Exchanges:
Calories: 166	Milk: 0.0
% Calories from Fat: 15	Vegetable: 2.0
Fat (gm): 2.8	Fruit: 0.0
Saturated Fat (gm): 1.5	Bread: 1.0
Cholesterol (mg): 5.6	Meat: 0.5
Sodium (mg): 603	Fat: 0.5
Protein (gm): 10.3	
Carbohydrate (gm): 24.6	

Spinach Soup

Surprise your guests at your next dinner party by adding an eight-ounce can of oysters to this recipe and calling it "Oysters Rockefeller Soup"!

1 14½-ounce can fat-free, sodium-reduced chicken stock
1 10-ounce package frozen chopped spinach, thawed
1 tablespoon dehydrated onion flakes
1 cup fat-free sour cream
Chopped chives for garnish (optional)

1. Combine chicken stock, spinach, and onion flakes in a saucepan and bring to a boil over medium-low heat. Remove from heat and allow to cool slightly. Pour mixture into a blender. Add sour cream and blend until smooth.

2. If you wish to serve soup hot, return it to saucepan and heat to desired temperature. Do not allow to boil. If you want to serve it cold, cover and refrigerate until well chilled. Garnish with chopped chives, if desired. (Makes 3 cups.)

SERVES 6 (½-cup servings)

Per Serving:	*Exchanges:*
Calories: 35	Milk: 0.0
% Calories from Fat: 2	Vegetable: 1.0
Fat (gm): 0.1	Fruit: 0.0
Saturated Fat (gm): 0	Bread: 0.0
Cholesterol (mg): 0	Meat: 0.0
Sodium (mg): 155	Fat: 0.0
Protein (gm): 4.3	
Carbohydrate (gm): 5.6	

Variation

Broccoli Soup: Substitute one 10-ounce package frozen broccoli for spinach.

Cheddar Cheese Soup

2 10¾-ounce cans low-fat cream of celery soup

1 14½-ounce can fat-free, sodium-reduced chicken stock

1 12-ounce can evaporated skim milk

4 ounces (1 cup) fat-reduced sharp Cheddar cheese, grated

2 tablespoons dehydrated onion flakes

1. Combine all ingredients in a saucepan and cook over low heat until cheese is melted. Do not allow to boil. Serve immediately. (Makes 6 cups.)

SERVES 6 (1-cup servings)

Per Serving:	*Exchanges:*
Calories: 117	Milk: 1.0
% Calories from Fat: 25	Vegetable: 0.0
Fat (gm): 3.3	Fruit: 0.0
Saturated Fat (gm): 1.4	Bread: 0.0
Cholesterol (mg): 13	Meat: 0.5
Sodium (mg): 527	Fat: 0.0
Protein (gm): 10.1	
Carbohydrate (gm): 11.5	

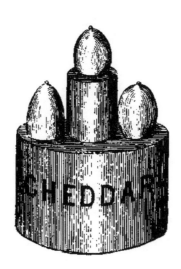

Crab Bisque

This soup is so surprisingly good that you will want to make it for dinner parties even when you aren't in a hurry. It can also be served cold, and it is a great addition to summer brunch and picnic menus.

1 10¾-ounce can reduced-sodium tomato soup

1 10¾-ounce can condensed green pea soup

1 12-ounce can evaporated skim milk

1 6½-ounce can crab, rinsed and drained

1 tablespoon corn oil margarine

¼ cup sherry

1. Combine all ingredients, except sherry and margarine, in a large saucepan, mix well, and heat to desired temperature. Add margarine and allow it to melt completely. Stir in sherry just before serving. (Makes 4½ cups.)

SERVES 6 (¾-cup servings)

Per Serving:	*Exchanges:*
Calories: 201	Milk: 0.5
% Calories from Fat: 22	Vegetable: 0.0
Fat (gm): 4.9	Fruit: 0.0
Saturated Fat (gm): 1.1	Bread: 1.0
Cholesterol (mg): 32.5	Meat: 1.0
Sodium (mg): 631	Fat: 0.5
Protein (gm): 13.8	
Carbohydrate (gm): 22.8	

Oyster Stew

You can use all other types of seafood, a well as oysters, in this basic recipe.

½ cup boiling water
⅓ cup Potato Buds
1 8-ounce bottle clam juice
⅛ teaspoon freshly ground black pepper
¼ teaspoon ground celery seed
1 12-ounce can evaporated skim milk
1 8-ounce can oysters, undrained

1. Combine boiling water and Potato Buds in a small bowl and whip until smooth. Set aside.

2. Combine all remaining ingredients, except oysters, in a saucepan and bring to boil over medium-low heat. Remove from heat and stir in potato mixture. Add oysters and all juice from can and mix well. Cover and allow to stand about 3 minutes. Serve immediately. (Makes 4 cups.)

SERVES 4 (1-cup servings)

Per Serving:
Calories: 118
% Calories from Fat: 12
Fat (gm): 1.6
Saturated Fat (gm): 0.5
Cholesterol (mg): 34
Sodium (mg): 239
Protein (gm): 11.3
Carbohydrate (gm): 13.9

Exchanges:
Milk: 1.0
Vegetable: 0.0
Fruit: 0.0
Bread: 0.0
Meat: 0.5
Fat: 0.0

Clam Chowder

1 tablespoon canola oil

1 medium onion, chopped, *or* 1½ cups frozen chopped onions

1 clove garlic, pressed or minced

1 2-ounce jar sliced pimiento, undrained

1 16½-ounce can low-sodium cream-style corn

1 10¾-ounce can condensed cream of potato soup

2 6½-ounce cans minced clams, undrained

1 12-ounce can evaporated skim milk

1 cup water

¼ teaspoon freshly ground black pepper

½ teaspoon dried basil, crushed

¼ teaspoon Liquid Smoke

2 tablespoons chopped fresh parsley (optional)

1. Heat oil in a large, heavy saucepan. Add onion and garlic and cook, covered, over low heat until onion is soft and translucent, about 10 minutes. Uncover and continue cooking, stirring frequently, until brown.

2. Add all remaining ingredients and continue to cook, covered, until hot, about 10 minutes. (Makes 8 cups.)

SERVES 6 (1⅓-cup servings)

Per Serving:	*Exchanges:*
Calories: 252	Milk: 0.5
% Calories from Fat: 17	Vegetable: 1.0
Fat (gm): 4.9	Fruit: 0.0
Saturated Fat (gm): 0.9	Bread: 1.0
Cholesterol (mg): 45.5	Meat: 2.0
Sodium (mg): 545	Fat: 0.0
Protein (gm): 22.4	
Carbohydrate (gm): 30.9	

Seafood Soup

This hearty, satisfying soup is a wonderfully easy one-dish meal. All you need to add is some crusty whole-grain or sourdough bread.

1 tablespoon extra-virgin olive oil

1 medium onion, chopped, *or* 1½ cups frozen chopped onions

2 garlic cloves, pressed or minced

2 6½-ounce cans chopped or minced clams, undrained

1 6-ounce can white crab, drained and rinsed (4½ ounces drained wt.)

1 6-ounce can shrimp, drained and rinsed (4½ ounces drained wt.)

1 10¾-ounce can sodium-reduced tomato soup

1 2-ounce jar sliced pimientos, undrained

1⅓ cups water

¼ cup chopped fresh parsley (optional)

¼ teaspoon salt

¼ teaspoon freshly ground black pepper

¼ teaspoon dried basil, crushed

¼ teaspoon dried oregano, crushed

⅛ teaspoon red pepper flakes

1. Heat oil in a large, heavy saucepan. Add onion and garlic and cook, covered, over low heat about 15 minutes or until onion is soft and translucent.

2. Stir in all remaining ingredients and continue to cook, covered, over low heat about 10 minutes or until hot. (Makes 6 cups.)

SERVES 4 (1½ cup servings)

Per Serving:
Calories: 315
% Calories from Fat: 23
Fat (gm): 7.9
Saturated Fat (gm): 1
Cholesterol (mg): 145.3
Sodium (mg): 425
Protein (gm): 39.5
Carbohydrate (gm): 19.7

Exchanges:
Milk: 0.0
Vegetable: 2.0
Fruit: 0.0
Bread: 0.5
Meat: 4.5
Fat: 0.0

Senegalese Soup

This is a really quick and easy version of the famous West African curried chicken soup, but it has all of the taste appeal of the original.

  6 teaspoons chopped raw almonds

  1 10¾-ounce can low-fat condensed cream of chicken soup

  1 12-ounce can evaporated skim milk

  1 3.9-ounce carton (½ cup) unsweetened applesauce

  ½ teaspoon curry powder, *or* to taste

  1 10-ounce can chunk white chicken in water, undrained

1. Put almonds in a skillet and cook over medium heat, stirring frequently, until well toasted. Set aside.

2. Combine all remaining ingredients, except chicken, in a blender and blend until satin smooth. Pour into a saucepan and bring to a boil over medium-low heat, stirring constantly.

3. Remove from heat and stir in chicken. Top each serving with a teaspoon of toasted almonds. (Makes 4½ cups.)

SERVES 6 (¾-cup servings)

Per Serving:	*Exchanges:*
Calories: 178	Milk: 0.5
% Calories from Fat: 34	Vegetable: 0.0
Fat (gm): 6.7	Fruit: 0.0
Saturated Fat (gm): 1.6	Bread: 0.5
Cholesterol (mg): 28.2	Meat: 1.5
Sodium (mg): 694	Fat: 0.5
Protein (gm): 16	
Carbohydrate (gm): 13.2	

Southwest Corn and Chicken Soup

1 tablespoon canola oil

1 small onion, finely chopped, *or* 1 cup frozen chopped onions

3 tablespoons all-purpose flour

½ teaspoon chili powder

¾ teaspoon ground cumin

1 14½-ounce can fat-free, sodium-reduced chicken stock, boiling

1 14½-ounce can chopped tomatoes, undrained

1 11-ounce can salt-free corn kernels, undrained

1 12-ounce can evaporated skim milk

1 10-ounce can chunk white chicken, undrained, flaked

1. Heat oil in a saucepan over medium-low heat. Add onion and cook, stirring frequently, until translucent. Add flour, chili powder, and cumin and cook, stirring constantly, 3 minutes.

2. Pour in boiling chicken stock and whisk until smooth. Add tomatoes and corn and mix well. Slowly stir in milk and heat to desired temperature. Do not allow to boil. Add chicken and mix well. (Makes 8 cups.)

SERVES 8 (1-cup servings)

Per Serving:
Calories: 162
% Calories from Fat: 27
Fat (gm): 5
Saturated Fat (gm): 1
Cholesterol (mg): 20.8
Sodium (mg): 391
Protein (gm): 13.7
Carbohydrate (gm): 16.4

Exchanges:
Milk: 0.5
Vegetable: 1.0
Fruit: 0.0
Bread: 0.5
Meat: 1.0
Fat: 0.0

Thai Chicken and Water Chestnut Soup

1 14½-ounce can fat-free, sodium-reduced chicken stock

2 cups water

1 tablespoon light brown sugar

½ teaspoon dried cilantro, crushed

3 tablespoons fish sauce

1 tablespoon rice vinegar

1 teaspoon chili paste

1 8-ounce can sliced water chestnuts, drained

1 10-ounce can chunk white chicken in water, undrained

1. Combine all ingredients, except water chestnuts and chicken, in a saucepan and bring to a boil. Reduce heat and simmer 10 minutes. Add water chestnuts and chicken. (Makes 6 cups.)

SERVES 6 (1-cup servings)

Per Serving:
Calories: 96
% Calories from Fat: 7
Fat (gm): 0.7
Saturated Fat (gm): 0
Cholesterol (mg): 2.3
Sodium (mg): 555
Protein (gm): 13.5
Carbohydrate (gm): 10.1

Exchanges:
Milk: 0.0
Vegetable: 1.0
Fruit: 0.0
Bread: 0.0
Meat: 1.5
Fat: 0.0

Turkey and Rice Soup

For a more economical soup, you can use one-half the amount of mushrooms called for in this recipe, or replace them with two four-ounce cans of sliced mushrooms, drained.

2 ounces (3 cups) dried mushrooms

2 14½-ounce cans fat-free, sodium-reduced chicken stock

¼ teaspoon ground celery seeds

½ cup uncooked instant brown rice

1 10-ounce can chunk turkey, undrained

2 tablespoons Madeira

1. Pour boiling water over dried mushrooms and allow to stand 20 minutes.

2. Bring chicken stock and celery seeds to a boil. Add rice and cook, covered, 5 minutes. Remove from heat, without removing lid, and allow to stand 5 more minutes.

3. While rice is cooking, drain mushrooms. Rinse well, picking over to remove any grit. Cut off stems and slice into ¼-in. strips. Add sliced mushrooms and turkey to rice, return to heat, and bring to a boil. Reduce heat to low and simmer, covered, 5 minutes. Add Madeira just before serving. (Makes 6 cups.)

SERVES 6 (1-cup servings)

Per Serving:	*Exchanges:*
Calories: 182	Milk: 0.0
% Calories from Fat: 20	Vegetable: 1.0
Fat (gm): 3.9	Fruit: 0.0
Saturated Fat (gm): 1.1	Bread: 1.0
Cholesterol (mg): 31.2	Meat: 1.5
Sodium (mg): 427	Fat: 0.0
Protein (gm): 16.6	
Carbohydrate (gm): 18.2	

THREE

Appetizers

AND

Salads

When I first started working on this book, I felt that creating really wonderful "pantry" salads would be the greatest challenge. Ironically, this has become the largest section in the book because I found so many combinations of ingredients that made exciting and deliciously different salads and appetizers. Many of these recipes are designed as entrees while others are better suited as appetizers or side dishes. Mix and match with available fresh products you may have on hand such as leftover fish, poultry, and meat, cooked vegetables, and fresh fruit. Or buy just the fresh vegetables and fruits you need in the salad bar section of your supermarket, all cleaned, chopped, and ready to use.

Sweet Dill Pickles ⑤ Artichoke Dip ⑤ Sweet Potato Dip or Sauce ⑤ Jelled Borsht Salad ⑤ Pink Party Salad ⑤ Tropical Fruit Salad ⑤ Potato Salad ⑤ Christmas Cabbage Salad Palm Hearts and Mandarin Oranges in Honeyed Mustard Dressing ⑤ Curried Tomato and Tofu Salad ⑤ Three-Bean Salad ⑤ Black Bean Salad ⑤ Roasted Sweet Pepper and Pinto Bean Salad ⑤ Green Bean Caesar Salad ⑤ Cannellini Bean Salad Dilled Tuna and Pasta Shell Salad ⑤ Mediterranean Tuna Salad Curried Chicken and Pineapple Salad ⑤ Taco Salad Caraway-Ham Coleslaw ⑤ Reuben Salad

Sweet Dill Pickles

If you find dill pickles too sour, and sweet pickles too sweet, here is the perfect compromise. These tasty treats are so good they can become habit forming. They also make a uniquely different host or hostess gift.

1 quart jar kosher dill pickles

1 cup sugar

1 teaspoon mustard seed

1 garlic clove, peeled, quartered

1. Drain pickles and cut into ½-inch slices. Return pickle slices to jar and add all remaining ingredients. Mix well and place in refrigerator. Allow to stand several days, turning jar daily. (Makes 3 cups.)

SERVES 12 (¼-cup servings)

Per Serving:	*Exchanges:*
Calories: 84	Milk: 0.0
% Calories from Fat: 1	Vegetable: 0.0
Fat (gm): 0.1	Fruit: 0.0
Saturated Fat (gm): 0	Bread: 1.0
Cholesterol (mg): 0	Meat: 0.0
Sodium (mg): 729	Fat: 0.0
Protein (gm): 0.1	
Carbohydrate (gm): 21.1	

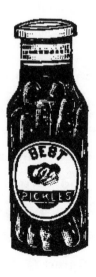

Artichoke Dip

This scrumptious, rich-tasting mixture has literally become my favorite dip. It can also be served as a vegetable side dish or chilled and served as a salad.

　　1 8½-ounce can artichoke hearts, drained, chopped

　　1 4-ounce can diced green chilies

　　¾ cup fat-free mayonnaise

　　3 ounces Parmesan cheese, grated (divided)

1. Preheat oven to 350°F.

2. Combine artichokes, chilies, mayonnaise, and all but 2 tablespoons cheese in an ovenproof bowl and mix well. Sprinkle remaining cheese evenly over top and bake in preheated oven 50 minutes or until the top is lightly browned. Serve warm, at room temperature, or cold as a dip, appetizer, vegetable side dish, or salad. (Makes 1½ cups.)

SERVES 24 (1-tablespoon servings)

Per Serving:	*Exchanges:*
Calories: 29	Milk: 0.0
% Calories from Fat: 34	Vegetable: 0.5
Fat (gm): 1.1	Fruit: 0.0
Saturated Fat (gm): 0.7	Bread: 0.0
Cholesterol (mg): 2.8	Meat: 0.0
Sodium (mg): 171	Fat: 0.5
Protein (gm): 1.9	
Carbohydrate (gm): 3.1	

Sweet Potato Dip or Sauce

There are about forty different varieties of sweet potatoes raised in this country, and they fall roughly into two categories: moist fleshed and dry fleshed. The ones that convert most of their starches to sugar during cooking and become sweet and soft are called "moist fleshed," or yam, varieties. Those that convert less starch and are therefore less sweet are called "dry fleshed." Although the sweeter varieties are often referred to as yams, they are not. True yams are starchy tropical vegetables rarely found in our markets. No one seems to know when or where this practice of calling sweet potatoes "yams" started, but it certainly is widespread and leads to lots of confusion. While I was working on this delicious and truly unusual dip, I had lots of fun asking people what they thought the ingredients were and very few guessed correctly. You can serve this dip with non-fat chips as a very low-fat appetizer or as a side dish with dinners. You can also thin it with a little non-fat milk for a wonderful sauce over pasta or rice.

    2 medium sweet potatoes (1½ lbs.)
    1 tablespoon dried marjoram, crushed
    ½ teaspoon ground nutmeg
    ¼ teaspoon salt
    ⅛ teaspoon freshly ground black pepper
    ⅛ teaspoon red pepper flakes
    1 tablespoon extra-virgin olive oil

1. Preheat oven to 400°F. Wash and dry sweet potatoes and poke holes in them with tines of a fork. Place them in a pan or on a baking sheet and bake in pre-heated oven 1 hour or until soft. Allow to cool until safe to handle. Remove and discard skins.

2. Put peeled sweet potatoes into a food processor. Add all other ingredients, except oil, and blend until satin smooth. Slowly add olive oil while processor is running. (Makes 1¾ cups.)

SERVES 14 (2-tablespoon servings)

Per Serving:	*Exchanges:*
Calories: 48	Milk: 0.0
% Calories from Fat: 19	Vegetable: 0.0
Fat (gm): 1	Fruit: 0.0
Saturated Fat (gm): 0.2	Bread: 0.5
Cholesterol (mg): 0	Meat: 0.0
Sodium (mg): 42	Fat: 0.0
Protein (gm): 0.7	
Carbohydrate (gm): 9.3	

Variation

Pumpkin Dip: Use one 16-ounce can solid-pack pumpkin in place of baked sweet potatoes. Add 2 tablespoons sugar and an additional ¼ teaspoon salt.

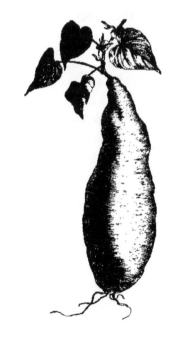

Jelled Borsht Salad

This is both an unusual and beautiful salad. You can also serve the jelled borsht in icers or bowls as a cold soup, and use the beets in other salads or in hot dishes.

1 16-ounce bottle of borsht with beets
2 envelopes unflavored gelatin
¼ cup light sour cream

1. Pour bottle of borsht with beets through a strainer to remove beets. Place beets in a covered container and refrigerate.

2. Soften gelatin in ¼ cup of strained borsht. Meanwhile, bring ¾ cup of borsht to a boil. Pour boiling borsht over softened gelatin and stir until completely dissolved; then add it to remaining borsht and mix well. Pour liquid into 8 x 8-in. baking dish and refrigerate until firm, about 3 hours.

3. To serve, spoon ¼ cup of beets onto each of 4 plates. Cut jelled borsht into small cubes, and spoon ¾ cup of the cubes on top of the beets. Top each serving with a tablespoon of sour cream.

SERVES 4

Per Serving:	*Exchanges:*
Calories: 67	Milk: 0.0
% Calories from Fat: 13	Vegetable: 2.0
Fat (gm): 0.9	Fruit: 0.0
Saturated Fat (gm): 0	Bread: 0.0
Cholesterol (mg): 4.7	Meat: 0.0
Sodium (mg): 325	Fat: 0.0
Protein (gm): 3.9	
Carbohydrate (gm): 10.4	

Pink Party Salad

This delightfully different shocking pink salad could also be called a "Way Out Waldorf." Just like the original Waldorf salad, it is a crunchy combination of apples, raisins, nuts, and other ingredients. However, unlike the original, the crunch comes primarily from canned water chestnuts rather than raw celery, and in place of raw apples I have used spiced crab apples from a jar. The advantage of this recipe is that all of the ingredients can be stored in your cupboard and the salad put together in minutes for a spur-of-the-moment festive meal.

½ cup raw almonds, chopped

¼ cup non-fat mayonnaise

¼ teaspoon curry powder

¼ teaspoon ground cinnamon

2 14-ounce jars spiced crab apples, drained, cored, chopped

1 8-ounce can water chestnuts, drained, chopped

¼ cup raisins

1. Place chopped almonds in a skillet and toast over medium heat. Watch carefully, as almonds burn easily. Set aside.

2. Combine mayonnaise, curry powder, and cinnamon in a bowl and mix well. Add all remaining ingredients, except toasted nuts, and mix well. Refrigerate until cold. Stir in toasted nuts just before serving. (Makes 2 cups.)

SERVES 4 (½-cup servings)

Per Serving:	*Exchanges:*
Calories: 359	Milk: 0.0
% Calories from Fat: 21	Vegetable: 2.0
Fat (gm): 8.6	Fruit: 4.0
Saturated Fat (gm): 0.8	Bread: 0.0
Cholesterol (mg): 0	Meat: 0.0
Sodium (mg): 198	Fat: 1.5
Protein (gm): 4.1	
Carbohydrate (gm): 70.4	

Tropical Fruit Salad

This refreshing combination of tropical fruits is wonderful served with cottage cheese as a vegetarian fruit salad or mixed with tuna or chicken. It also makes a delicious dessert.

1 10½ -ounce can mandarin orange sections in juice

1 20-ounce can pineapple chunks in juice, drained

1 11-ounce can lychees, rinsed, drained

¼ cup Grand Marnier, *or* any orange liqueur

½ cup fat-free sour cream

2 tablespoons crushed macadamia nuts for garnish (optional)

1. Combine all fruit in a large bowl. Add Grand Marnier and mix well. Cover and refrigerate until chilled. Just before serving, fold sour cream into the fruit mixture. Garnish each serving with a teaspoon of crushed macadamia nuts, if desired. (Makes 3 cups.)

SERVES 6 (½-cup servings)

Per Serving:	*Exchanges:*
Calories: 157	Milk: 0.0
% Calories from Fat: 2	Vegetable: 0.0
Fat (gm): 0.5	Fruit: 2.0
Saturated Fat (gm): 0	Bread: 0.0
Cholesterol (mg): 0	Meat: 0.0
Sodium (mg): 16	Fat: 0.5
Protein (gm): 2.6	
Carbohydrate (gm): 33.7	

Potato Salad

If you're putting together a spur-of-the-moment picnic and want a really quick-and-easy potato salad, here is the perfect recipe. From start to finish, it takes about seven minutes.

Dressing

⅓ cup fat-free mayonnaise

1 teaspoon cider vinegar

1 tablespoon brown mustard

¼ teaspoon salt

¼ teaspoon freshly ground black pepper

½ teaspoon celery seed

Salad

2 15-ounce cans new potatoes, drained, diced

½ cup chopped onion

1 4-ounce jar sliced pimiento

1. Combine all dressing ingredients in a large bowl and mix well. Add all salad ingredients and again mix well. Cover and refrigerate several hours (if possible) before serving (Makes 4 cups.)

SERVES 8 (½-cup servings)

Per Serving:	*Exchanges:*
Calories: 82	Milk: 0.0
% Calories from Fat: 5	Vegetable: 0.5
Fat (gm): 0.5	Fruit: 0.0
Saturated Fat (gm): 0.1	Bread: 1.0
Cholesterol (mg): 0	Meat: 0.0
Sodium (mg): 499	Fat: 0.0
Protein (gm): 1.9	
Carbohydrate (gm): 18.4	

Christmas Cabbage Salad

Because the ingredients in this recipe are the traditional holiday colors, red, green, and white, I call it a Christmas salad. Also, it is perfect for holiday entertaining because it can be made ahead of time and works wonderfully well for buffets.

3 cups finely chopped red cabbage

1 8½-ounce can sweet green peas, drained

¾ cup fat-free ranch dressing

1. Combine all ingredients in a large bowl and mix well. Cover and refrigerate several hours before serving. (Makes 3 cups.)

SERVES 6 (½-cup servings)

Per Serving:
Calories: 69
% Calories from Fat: 3
Fat (gm): 0.2
Saturated Fat (gm): 0
Cholesterol (mg): 0
Sodium (mg): 392
Protein (gm): 2.3
Carbohydrate (gm): 13.2

Exchanges:
Milk: 0.0
Vegetable: 1.0
Fruit: 0.0
Bread: 0.5
Meat: 0.0
Fat: 0.0

Palm Hearts and Mandarin Oranges in Honeyed Mustard Dressing

This salad is just as pretty as it is delicious. Also, the dressing can be used on greens or other fruits and vegetables.

Dressing

> ¼ cup fat-free mayonnaise
>
> 2 tablespoons honeyed mustard
>
> 2 tablespoons lime juice
>
> 1 teaspoon lime zest
>
> 2 teaspoons extra-virgin olive oil

Salad

> 1 8-ounce can palm hearts, cut lengthwise into thin strips
>
> 1 10½-ounce can mandarin oranges in juice

1. Combine all dressing ingredients, except oil, in a small bowl and mix well. Whisk in oil and set aside.

2. Arrange strips of palm hearts and mandarin orange sections on 4 plates. Drizzle about 2 tablespoons dressing over each serving.

SERVES 4

Per Serving:	*Exchanges:*
Calories: 127	Milk: 0.0
% Calories from Fat: 20	Vegetable: 0.0
Fat (gm): 2.9	Fruit: 0.5
Saturated Fat (gm): 0.4	Bread: 1.0
Cholesterol (mg): 0	Meat: 0.0
Sodium (mg): 302	Fat: 0.5
Protein (gm): 2.5	
Carbohydrate (gm): 24.1	

Curried Tomato and Tofu Salad

This delightfully different vegetarian salad is even better if it is made several hours before serving. It is also a wonderful filling for pita pocket sandwiches.

2 tablespoons fat-free mayonnaise

1 tablespoon sodium-reduced soy sauce

⅛ teaspoon red pepper flakes

¼ teaspoon freshly ground black pepper

¼ teaspoon ground ginger

½ teaspoon turmeric

1 teaspoon curry powder

½ cup chopped onions, *or* scallions

1 14½-ounce can chopped tomatoes, drained

1 10½-ounce package silken-firm tofu, diced

Fresh cilantro leaves for garnish (optional)

1. Combine all ingredients, except tomatoes and tofu, in a bowl and mix well. Add remaining ingredients and again mix well. Cover and refrigerate several hours before serving. Garnish with cilantro, if desired. (Makes 3 cups.)

SERVES 6 (½-cup servings)

Per Serving:	*Exchanges:*
Calories: 57	Milk: 0.0
% Calories from Fat: 20	Vegetable: 1.5
Fat (gm): 1.3	Fruit: 0.0
Saturated Fat (gm): 0	Bread: 0.0
Cholesterol (mg): 0	Meat: 0.5
Sodium (mg): 295	Fat: 0.0
Protein (gm): 5.1	
Carbohydrate (gm): 7	

Three-Bean Salad

This is the easiest and fastest version of this classic picnic salad that I know of, and it is very good! If you want a little "zippier" taste, add some chopped onion.

¾ cup fat-free Italian salad dressing

¼ cup sugar

1 16-ounce can cut green beans, drained

1 16-ounce can cut wax beans, drained

1 15-ounce can dark red kidney beans, drained

½ cup chopped onion (optional)

1. Combine salad dressing and sugar in a large bowl and stir until sugar has dissolved. Add all drained beans and mix well. Cover and refrigerate several hours or overnight before serving. Garnish with onions, if desired. (Makes 3½ cups.)

SERVES 7 (½-cup servings)

Per Serving:	Exchanges:
Calories: 118	Milk: 0.0
% Calories from Fat: 4	Vegetable: 2.0
Fat (gm): 0.6	Fruit: 0.0
Saturated Fat (gm): 0	Bread: 1.0
Cholesterol (mg): 0	Meat: 0.0
Sodium (mg): 799	Fat: 0.0
Protein (gm): 6.4	
Carbohydrate (gm): 26	

Black Bean Salad

This spicy salad is perfect for picnics and tailgate parties. It can also be turned into a delicious dip to serve with fat-free tortilla chips just by pureeing the beans before combining them with the cooked ingredients.

1 medium onion, chopped, *or* 1½ cups frozen chopped onions

1 clove garlic, pressed or minced

1 7-ounce can diced green chilies

¼ teaspoon salt

½ teaspoon freshly ground black pepper

½ teaspoon ground cumin

1½ teaspoons chili powder

2 15-ounce cans black beans, drained

1. Combine onion and garlic in a heavy saucepan and cook, covered, over low heat 10 minutes or until onion is translucent, adding a little water if necessary to prevent scorching. Add diced chilies, salt, pepper, cumin, and chili powder and cook 3 more minutes. Add drained beans and mix well. (Makes 4 cups.)

SERVES 8 (½-cup servings)

Per Serving:	*Exchanges:*
Calories: 100	Milk: 0.0
% Calories from Fat: 8	Vegetable: 1.0
Fat (gm): 1.1	Fruit: 0.0
Saturated Fat (gm): 0	Bread: 1.0
Cholesterol (mg): 0	Meat: 0.0
Sodium (mg): 695	Fat: 0.0
Protein (gm): 9.1	
Carbohydrate (gm): 21.4	

Roasted Sweet Pepper and Pinto Bean Salad

Cooking the ingredients in this salad really intensifies their tastes. It can also be served as a hot vegetable side dish or combined with canned tuna or chicken for a hot or cold entree.

  1 tablespoon extra-virgin olive oil
  1 garlic clove, pressed or minced
  1 medium onion, chopped, *or* 1½ cups frozen chopped onions
  ¾ teaspoon dried oregano, crushed
  ¾ teaspoon dried basil, crushed
  ¼ teaspoon freshly ground black pepper
  ⅛ teaspoon red pepper flakes
  2 7-ounce cans roasted red sweet peppers, drained, sliced
  1 15-ounce can pinto beans, drained

1. Heat oil in a large skillet over medium heat. Add garlic and cook until it sizzles. Add onion and all ingredients, except roasted peppers and beans, and cook, stirring frequently, until onion is translucent, about 5 minutes. Stir in sliced peppers and drained beans and continue to cook 2 more minutes.

2. Remove from heat and allow to come to room temperature before serving; or refrigerate and serve cold. (Makes 2⅔ cups.)

SERVES 4 (⅔-cup servings)

Per Serving:	*Exchanges:*
Calories: 187	Milk: 0.0
% Calories from Fat: 20	Vegetable: 2.0
Fat (gm): 4.5	Fruit: 0.0
Saturated Fat (gm): 0.5	Bread: 1.5
Cholesterol (mg): 0	Meat: 0.0
Sodium (mg): 391	Fat: 0.5
Protein (gm): 9.3	
Carbohydrate (gm): 32.2	

Green Bean Caesar Salad

This egg-free, pantry version of a Caesar salad is made with thawed green beans rather than romaine lettuce. Try adding leftover poultry or meat for an entree salad, and serve it with whole-grain bread, pasta, rice, or beans to bring the fat calories for the meal down to 30 percent.

2 tablespoons extra-virgin olive oil

1 garlic clove, pressed or minced

1 16-ounce bag frozen French cut green beans, thawed

2 tablespoons lemon juice

1 tablespoon Worcestershire sauce

1 tablespoon red wine vinegar

1½ teaspoons anchovy paste

¼ teaspoon freshly ground black pepper

½ cup (2 ounces) Parmesan cheese, shredded

1½ cups Croutons, see page 126

1. Combine oil and garlic in skillet and cook over medium heat just until garlic sizzles. Add beans and cook, stirring constantly, 3 minutes. Remove from heat and stir in all remaining ingredients, except croutons, and toss thoroughly. Serve warm or refrigerate until cold. Top each serving with ¼ cup croutons, if desired. (Makes 4 cups.)

SERVES 6 (⅔-cup servings)

Per Serving:	*Exchanges:*
Calories: 137	Milk: 0.0
% Calories from Fat: 48	Vegetable: 1.0
Fat (gm): 7.6	Fruit: 0.0
Saturated Fat (gm): 2.3	Bread: 0.5
Cholesterol (mg): 6.6	Meat: 0.0
Sodium (mg): 278	Fat: 1.5
Protein (gm): 6	
Carbohydrate (gm): 12.8	

Cannellini Bean Salad

This is a terrific salad for picnics and tailgate parties because it contains no animal protein and is therefore safe to leave unrefrigerated for hours. Also, it is better tasting served at room temperature than cold.

1 tablespoon extra-virgin olive oil

1 tablespoon lemon juice

¼ teaspoon freshly ground black pepper

⅛ teaspoon red pepper flakes

½ teaspoon dried oregano, crushed

1 garlic clove, pressed or minced

¼ cup chopped onion

1 14½-ounce can chopped tomatoes, drained

1 15-ounce can cannellini beans, drained

2 tablespoons chopped fresh parsley (optional)

1. Combine olive oil, lemon juice, pepper, pepper flakes, oregano, and garlic in a bowl and mix well. Add onion, drained tomatoes, beans, and (optional) parsley and again mix well. (Makes 3 cups.)

SERVES 4 (¾-cup servings)

Per Serving:	*Exchanges:*
Calories: 133	Milk: 0.0
% Calories from Fat: 23	Vegetable: 2.0
Fat (gm): 4.4	Fruit: 0.0
Saturated Fat (gm): 0.5	Bread: 1.0
Cholesterol (mg): 0	Meat: 0.0
Sodium (mg): 377	Fat: 0.5
Protein (gm): 8.8	
Carbohydrate (gm): 24.1	

Dilled Tuna and Pasta Shell Salad

You can make this recipe with any type of pasta, but the shells make a great look-ing salad for parties. Also, the addition of pimiento makes a more colorful salad.

¼ cup fat-free mayonnaise

¼ cup fat-free plain yogurt

1 tablespoon rice vinegar

½ teaspoon dried dill weed, crushed

¼ teaspoon dried tarragon, crushed

⅛ teaspoon salt

⅛ teaspoon freshly ground black pepper

2 cups cooked pasta shells

1 6-ounce can solid-pack white tuna in water, drained, flaked

½ cup frozen peas, blanched, drained

1 2-ounce jar sliced pimientos, drained (optional)

1. Combine all ingredients, except pasta, tuna, and peas, in a bowl and mix well. Add remaining ingredients and again mix well. (Makes 3 cups.)

SERVES 4 (¾-cup servings)

Per Serving:	*Exchanges:*
Calories: 195	Milk: 0.0
% Calories from Fat: 8	Vegetable: 0.0
Fat (gm): 1.6	Fruit: 0.0
Saturated Fat (gm): 0.4	Bread: 1.5
Cholesterol (mg): 18.1	Meat: 1.5
Sodium (mg): 456	Fat: 0.0
Protein (gm): 16.8	
Carbohydrate (gm): 27.1	

Mediterranean Tuna Salad

I ordered this light and delicious salad at Capers in Seattle when I was there last summer, and I liked it so much that I asked the owner, Lisa Meyers, for her recipe. It is wonderful served on fresh greens or mixed with pasta, rice, or beans.

1 12-ounce can solid-pack white tuna in water, drained, flaked

¼ cup lemon juice

½ teaspoon lemon zest (optional)

2 tablespoons capers

12 kalamata pitted olives, thinly sliced

1. Combine all ingredients in a bowl and mix well. (Makes 1⅓ cups.)

SERVES 4 (⅓-cup servings)

Per Serving:
Calories: 147
% Calories from Fat: 22
Fat (gm): 3.6
Saturated Fat (gm): 0.8
Cholesterol (mg): 35.8
Sodium (mg): 536
Protein (gm): 23.4
Carbohydrate (gm): 4.7

Exchanges:
Milk: 0.0
Vegetable: 0.0
Fruit: 0.0
Bread: 0.0
Meat: 3.0
Fat: 0.0

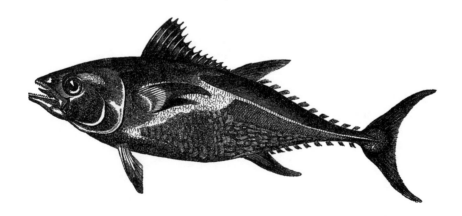

Curried Chicken and Pineapple Salad

This salad is also good made with tuna, and you can substitute water chestnuts for the bamboo shoots if you prefer a little more crunch in your salad. I suggest serving this salad with fat-free cinnamon rice cakes, which are not only a perfect taste accompaniment but also will lower the percentage of total fat calories in the meal.

¼ cup raw almonds, chopped

⅓ cup fat-free mayonnaise

1¼ teaspoons curry powder

¼ teaspoon ground ginger

⅛ teaspoon red pepper flakes

3 tablespoons mango chutney

1 8-ounce can pineapple chunks in natural juice, drained

1 10-ounce can white chicken

1 8-ounce can sliced bamboo shoots, drained

1. Put almonds in a skillet and cook over medium heat until well toasted. Set aside.

2. Combine all ingredients, except pineapple, chicken, and bamboo shoots, in a large bowl and mix well. Add all remaining ingredients and again mix well. Cover and refrigerate until cold before serving.

3. To serve, spoon ¾ cup of salad onto each of 4 plates. Top each serving with 1 tablespoon toasted almonds. (Makes 3 cups.)

SERVES 4 (¾-cup servings)

Per Serving:	*Exchanges:*
Calories: 258	Milk: 0.0
% Calories from Fat: 35	Vegetable: 2.0
Fat (gm): 10.3	Fruit: 1.0
Saturated Fat (gm): 2	Bread: 0.0
Cholesterol (mg): 38.9	Meat: 2.0
Sodium (mg): 619	Fat: 1.0
Protein (gm): 18.4	
Carbohydrate (gm): 24.2	

Taco Salad

In place of the fat-free chips called for in this recipe, you can serve hot corn tortillas on the side and let your guests make soft tacos by filling them with salad. Be sure to drain the salsa, as this is the major source of sodium in this recipe, which is not recommended for those on a strict low-sodium diet.

1½ cups chunky salsa, thoroughly drained

⅛ teaspoon ground cumin

1 11-ounce can salt-free corn kernels, drained

1 10-ounce can white chunk chicken, drained

2 ounces (½ cup) fat-reduced sharp Cheddar cheese, grated (divided)

4 ounces (4 cups) fat-free tortilla chips

¼ cup light sour cream

1. Combine salsa and cumin in a bowl and mix well. Stir in corn, chicken, and ¼ cup of the cheese. Spoon 1 cup of mixture onto each of 4 plates. Arrange 1 cup of chips around each serving, and sprinkle with 1 tablespoon cheese. Top each serving with 1 tablespoon sour cream. (Makes 4 cups.)

SERVES 4 (1-cup servings)

Per Serving:	*Exchanges:*
Calories: 343	Milk: 0.0
% Calories from Fat: 27	Vegetable: 0.0
Fat (gm): 10.4	Fruit: 0.0
Saturated Fat (gm): 2.6	Bread: 2.5
Cholesterol (mg): 53.8	Meat: 2.5
Sodium (mg): 1246	Fat: 0.5
Protein (gm): 24.2	
Carbohydrate (gm): 38.2	

Caraway-Ham Coleslaw

This is a super coleslaw with or without the ham. You can also substitute canned chicken or corned beef for the ham or use up any leftover meat you may have on hand.

¼ cup fat-free mayonnaise

1 tablespoon herbed vinegar

2 tablespoons Dijon mustard

1 teaspoon sugar

⅛ teaspoon salt

⅛ teaspoon freshly ground black pepper

½ teaspoon caraway seeds

1 8-ounce package (3 cups) coleslaw

1 5-ounce can extra-lean chunk ham, flaked

1. Combine all ingredients, except coleslaw and ham, in a bowl and mix well. Add remaining ingredients and again mix well. (Makes 3 cups.)

SERVES 6 (½-cup servings)

Per Serving:	*Exchanges:*
Calories: 58	Milk: 0.0
% Calories from Fat: 24	Vegetable: 1.0
Fat (gm): 1.6	Fruit: 0.0
Saturated Fat (gm): 0.4	Bread: 0.0
Cholesterol (mg): 7.1	Meat: 0.5
Sodium (mg): 513	Fat: 0.0
Protein (gm): 5.8	
Carbohydrate (gm): 5.4	

Reuben Salad

This salad has all of the fabulous flavors of the famous sandwich for which it is named. If you are making this salad ahead of time, cover and refrigerate it without adding the crumbs. If you are serving it immediately, you might want to toss the salad instead of layering it, and then top each serving with two tablespoons of crumbs.

Dressing

> 1 8-ounce carton fat-free sour cream
>
> ¼ cup chili sauce
>
> 2 tablespoons dehydrated onion flakes
>
> 1 tablespoon honey

Salad

> 1 8-ounce bag coleslaw
>
> 1 14½-ounce can sauerkraut, drained, rinsed
>
> ¼ cup chopped parsley (optional)
>
> 1 12-ounce can corned beef, flaked
>
> 6 ounces (1½ cups) fat-reduced Swiss cheese, diced
>
> ½ teaspoon caraway seeds
>
> 1 cup toasted breadcrumbs

1. Combine all dressing ingredients in bowl and mix well.

2. Line bottom of large bowl with ½ of coleslaw. Add sauerkraut and (optional) parsley. Spread corned beef evenly over top of sauerkraut. Sprinkle cheese over meat and top with remaining coleslaw.

3. Spread dressing over top of salad. Sprinkle caraway seeds and toasted breadcrumbs evenly over dressing. (Makes 10 cups.)

SERVES 10 (1-cup servings)

Per Serving:	Exchanges:
Calories: 214	Milk: 0.0
% Calories from Fat: 33	Vegetable: 2.0
Fat (gm): 7.6	Fruit: 0.0
Saturated Fat (gm): 3.5	Bread: 0.5
Cholesterol (mg): 38.3	Meat: 1.5
Sodium (mg): 940	Fat: 0.5
Protein (gm): 16.6	
Carbohydrate (gm): 18.7	

FOUR

Meatless Meals

*I am calling this section meatless rather than vegetarian because
I have used chicken stock in some of the recipes. However, if you wish to
use these recipes for strictly vegetarian meal planning, just substitute
vegetable stock. I have also included a few recipes for vegetable side dishes
that can be mixed and matched with the other recipes in the book.*

Quesadillas ❦ Bean Burritos ❦ Pinto Bean and Pea Pasta
with Dried Tomato Sauce ❦ Eggs Foo Yung ❦ Fettuccine
with Shiitake Mushrooms ❦ Fuselli with Green Beans
Moroccan Chickpeas and Couscous ❦ Spicy Lentil Stew
Asparagus au Gratin ❦ Hawaiian Green Beans ❦ Honeyed
Beets ❦ Herbed Scalloped Potatoes ❦ Tuscan Potatoes

Quesadillas

You can use your own imagination, and what you have on hand, to jazz up these tasty Mexican melted cheese sandwiches. You can use other cheeses or combinations such as sharp Cheddar with the Jack cheese. You can also add a little fish, poultry, or meat to the filling. Always serve your favorite salsa on the side.

    4 fat-free whole wheat tortillas

    6 ounces (1½ cups) fat-reduced Monterey Jack cheese, shredded

    1 4-ounce can diced green chilies

1. Heat a non-stick skillet sprayed with a non-stick vegetable cooking spray over medium-low heat. Place a tortilla in skillet and sprinkle ¼ cup plus 2 tablespoons cheese evenly over the top.

2. When cheese melts, sprinkle 2 tablespoons diced chilies over the top. Fold tortilla in half and cut into 3 pie-shaped wedges.

SERVES 4

Per Serving:	*Exchanges:*
Calories: 198	Milk: 0.0
% Calories from Fat: 32	Vegetable: 0.5
Fat (gm): 7.6	Fruit: 0.0
Saturated Fat (gm): 4.6	Bread: 1.0
Cholesterol (mg): 30.4	Meat: 2.0
Sodium (mg): 951	Fat: 0.0
Protein (gm): 16.8	
Carbohydrate (gm): 18.8	

Bean Burritos

This is the basic recipe for these popular and easy-to-make Mexican "sandwiches." For variety you can add other ingredients to the beans such as leftover cooked vegetables, grated cheese, or sautéed onions. Burritos are good served with light or fat-free sour cream and salsa.

10 fat-free whole wheat tortillas (17½-ounce package)
2 16-ounce cans vegetarian refried beans
1 4-ounce can diced green chilies
5 ounces fat-reduced sharp Cheddar cheese, grated (optional)

1. Preheat oven to 350°F. Wrap tortillas in foil and place them in preheated oven for 10 minutes or until warm and pliable.

2. While tortillas are warming, combine beans and chilies in a saucepan and cook over medium heat, stirring frequently, until hot.

3. To make burritos, spoon ⅓ cup bean mixture onto lower half of each tortilla. Sprinkle with 2 tablespoons cheese, if desired. Fold tortilla, envelope style, around bean mixture.

SERVES 10

Per Serving:
Calories: 184
% Calories from Fat: 4
Fat (gm): 0.9
Saturated Fat (gm): 0.3
Cholesterol (mg): 7.4
Sodium (mg): 901
Protein (gm): 9.7
Carbohydrate (gm): 39.6

Exchanges:
Milk: 0.0
Vegetable: 3.0
Fruit: 0.0
Bread: 1.5
Meat: 0.0
Fat: 0.0

Pinto Bean and Pea Pasta with Dried Tomato Sauce

1 10¾-ounce can low-fat cream of chicken soup

⅔ cup Sonoma dried tomato bits

¼ teaspoon freshly ground black pepper

2 garlic cloves, pressed or minced, *or* ¼ teaspoon garlic powder

1½ teaspoons Italian herb blend, crushed

½ teaspoon Liquid Smoke

1 10-ounce package (2 cups) frozen peas, thawed

1 16-ounce can pinto beans, drained

8 ounces cooked rigatoni pasta, cooked *al dente* according to package directions

½ cup freshly grated Parmesan cheese (optional)

1. Combine soup and 1 soup can of water, *or* (optional) skim milk, in large saucepan. Add dried tomatoes, pepper, garlic, Italian herbs, and Liquid Smoke and bring to boil over medium heat. Reduce heat to low and simmer, stirring frequently, 5 minutes.

2. Stir in peas and pinto beans and heat through. Remove from heat and stir in cooked pasta. Sprinkle (optional) Parmesan over each serving.

SERVES 4 (1¾-cup servings)

Per Serving:	*Exchanges:*
Calories: 426	Milk: 0.0
% Calories from Fat: 6	Vegetable: 0.0
Fat (gm): 3	Fruit: 0.0
Saturated Fat (gm): 0.2	Bread: 5.5
Cholesterol (mg): 1.7	Meat: 0.0
Sodium (mg): 812	Fat: 0.5
Protein (gm): 20.5	
Carbohydrate (gm): 82.9	

Eggs Foo Yung

If you don't have any fresh green onion tops to add to these little Chinese omelettes, use a tablespoon of dehydrated dried onions to replace them.

½ cup water

2 teaspoons cornstarch

2 tablespoons low-sodium soy sauce

1½ teaspoons cider vinegar

¼ teaspoon salt

1 teaspoon sugar

1½ cups non-fat liquid egg substitute

1 16-ounce can bean sprouts, drained

½ cup finely chopped green onion tops (optional)

2 6½-ounce cans shrimp, drained, rinsed

1. Combine water and cornstarch in a saucepan and stir until completely dissolved. Stir in soy sauce, vinegar, salt, and sugar. Cook over medium low heat, stirring constantly, until thickened. Set sauce aside to spoon over patties.

2. Combine all remaining ingredients in bowl and mix well. Spray a large non-stick skillet with non-stick vegetable cooking spray and heat over medium heat until drops of water dance on surface. Spoon mixture into hot skillet as you would pancakes, a rounded ¼ cup at a time. When lightly browned, turn patties and brown other side. Reduce heat to low and continue cooking 5 more minutes or until completely done. Serve Egg Foo Yung with sauce spooned over top.

SERVES 6 (2-patty servings)

Per Serving:	*Exchanges:*
Calories: 117	Milk: 0.0
% Calories from Fat: 10	Vegetable: 1.0
Fat (gm): 1.4	Fruit: 0.0
Saturated Fat (gm): 0.3	Bread: 0.0
Cholesterol (mg): 106.5	Meat: 2.0
Sodium (mg): 475	Fat: 0.0
Protein (gm): 20.8	
Carbohydrate (gm): 5.5	

Fettuccine with Shiitake Mushrooms

Dried mushrooms are wonderful to keep in the pantry because they are so versatile and add such panache to many otherwise plain recipes.

3 ounces (4½ cups) dried shiitake mushrooms
2 teaspoons olive oil
2 cloves garlic, pressed or minced
2 tablespoons minced shallot, *or* onion
½ cup water
¼ cup dry skim milk powder
¼ cup sherry
1 teaspoon sodium-reduced soy sauce
⅛ teaspoon freshly ground black pepper, *or* to taste
8 ounces dry fettuccine pasta (4 cups cooked)
Finely chopped parsley for garnish (optional)

1. To reconstitute the dried mushrooms, cover them with boiling water and allow to stand 20 minutes. Drain and rinse to remove any grit. Then cut off stems, using scissors, and slice into ½-in. strips.

2. Heat oil in a heavy skillet. Add garlic and shallots and cook, over medium heat, stirring frequently, until shallots are translucent, about 3 minutes. Reduce heat to low and add sliced shiitakes. Cook, stirring frequently, 15 minutes.

3. Combine water and milk powder, stir until completely dissolved, and add to pan. Then add sherry, soy sauce, and pepper and simmer 10 minutes.

4. Cook the fettuccine *al dente* according to package directions. Drain thoroughly and place in a warm bowl. Spoon sauce over top and garnish with chopped parsley, if desired.

SERVES 3

Per Serving:	*Exchanges:*
Calories: 428	Milk: 0.0
% Calories from Fat: 11	Vegetable: 1.0
Fat (gm): 5.5	Fruit: 0.0
Saturated Fat (gm): 0.8	Bread: 5.0
Cholesterol (mg): 1	Meat: 0.0
Sodium (mg): 103	Fat: 1.0
Protein (gm): 15.4	
Carbohydrate (gm): 77.1	

Fuselli with Green Beans

This easy and delicious pasta dish can be made with other canned vegetables or any leftover cooked vegetable. It is also good with either canned or leftover fish, poultry, or meat added to it.

8 ounces dry fuselli pasta (4 cups cooked)

1 tablespoon extra-virgin olive oil

1 garlic clove, pressed or minced

⅛ teaspoon freshly ground black pepper

⅛ teaspoon red pepper flakes

1 14½-ounce can French-cut green beans, drained

½ cup shredded Parmesan cheese

1. Cook pasta *al dente* according to package directions.

2. While pasta is cooking, combine oil, garlic, pepper and red pepper flakes in a skillet and cook over medium heat until garlic starts to sizzle. Stir in drained green beans and cook until hot.

3. In a large bowl, combine drained pasta, bean mixture, and cheese; toss thoroughly. Serve immediately.

SERVES 4 (1-cup servings)

Per Serving:	*Exchanges:*
Calories: 303	Milk: 0.0
% Calories from Fat: 26	Vegetable: 1.0
Fat (gm): 8.8	Fruit: 0.0
Saturated Fat (gm): 3.1	Bread: 2.5
Cholesterol (mg): 9.9	Meat: 0.5
Sodium (mg): 499	Fat: 1.5
Protein (gm): 14.1	
Carbohydrate (gm): 42.3	

Moroccan Chickpeas and Couscous

This rather exotically seasoned combination of ingredients provides a complete protein because it includes both a legume and a grain. It is a moist mixture that can easily be pressed into a mold and turned out onto the serving plate, hot or cold. I like it best served at room temperature surrounded by either fresh orange slices or juice-packed Mandarin orange sections.

1 medium onion, chopped, *or* 1½ frozen chopped onions

1 14½-ounce can fat-free, sodium-reduced chicken stock

¾ cup water

1 14½-ounce can chopped tomatoes, undrained

1 16-ounce can chickpeas (garbanzo beans), drained

1¼ teaspoons ground coriander

1 teaspoon ground cumin

1 10-ounce box couscous

1. Combine onion and ¼ cup chicken stock in a saucepan and cook over medium-low heat until onion is soft and translucent. Add all ingredients, except couscous, and bring to a boil. Reduce heat to low and simmer, covered, 10 minutes.

2. Add couscous and mix well. Cover tightly and remove from heat. Allow to stand 5 minutes or until liquid has all been absorbed.

SERVES 8 (1-cup servings)

Per Serving:	*Exchanges:*
Calories: 211	Milk: 0.0
% Calories from Fat: 7	Vegetable: 0.0
Fat (gm): 1.7	Fruit: 0.0
Saturated Fat (gm): 0.2	Bread: 3.0
Cholesterol (mg): 0	Meat: 0.0
Sodium (mg): 390	Fat: 0.0
Protein (gm): 8.9	
Carbohydrate (gm): 40.6	

Spicy Lentil Stew

You can serve this versatile, tangy dish hot or at room temperature as a side dish or cold as a lentil salad. For an entree, top each serving with cheese, a suggested optional ingredient, or add a can of tuna or chicken just before serving.

1 medium onion, chopped, *or* 1½ cups frozen chopped onions

2 garlic cloves, pressed or minced

1 cup dry lentils

1 14½-ounce can fat-free, sodium-reduced chicken stock

¼ cup water

1 14½-ounce can chopped Italian-style tomatoes, undrained

1 4-ounce jar spicy sliced pimientos

¼ teaspoon freshly ground black pepper

1 teaspoon dried thyme, crushed

4 ounces (1 cup) fat-reduced sharp Cheddar, or Monterey Jack cheese, grated (optional)

1. Combine onion and garlic in a heavy saucepan and cook, covered, over low heat about 15 minutes or until onion is soft and translucent. Add lentils and stock and bring to a boil. Reduce heat to low and simmer 30 minutes or until lentils are tender and all liquid has been absorbed.

2. Add all remaining ingredients, except cheese, and simmer 10 minutes. Top each serving with ¼ cup (optional) grated cheese and allow it to melt.

SERVES 4 (1¼-cup servings)

Per Serving:	*Exchanges:*
Calories: 227	Milk: 0.0
% Calories from Fat: 6	Vegetable: 2.0
Fat (gm): 1.6	Fruit: 0.0
Saturated Fat (gm): 0.2	Bread: 2.0
Cholesterol (mg): 0	Meat: 0.5
Sodium (mg): 333	Fat: 0.0
Protein (gm): 17.2	
Carbohydrate (gm): 39.9	

Asparagus au Gratin

This easy-to-make and delicious combination of asparagus and cheese can either be served as a vegetable side dish or, in larger servings, as an entree.

1 15-ounce can asparagus spears

1 4-ounce bag (about 1½ cups) unsalted, fat-free potato chips, crushed

1 10¾-ounce can low-fat cream of mushroom soup

4 ounces (1 cup) fat-reduced sharp Cheddar cheese, grated

½ cup breadcrumbs

¼ teaspoon paprika

1. Preheat oven to 350°F. Spray a 7 x 11-in. baking dish with non-stick vegetable cooking spray. Drain asparagus, reserving ½ cup liquid from can.

2. Arrange asparagus spears on bottom of prepared dish. Top with ½ of crumbled potato chips. Spread ½ of soup over potato chips. Top soup with remaining potato chips. Add asparagus liquid to remaining soup and pour evenly over potato chips.

3. Sprinkle top of dish with cheese, breadcrumbs, and paprika. Bake in preheated oven about 30 minutes or until bubbly.

SERVES 6 (⅔-cup servings)

Per Serving:	*Exchanges:*
Calories: 127	Milk: 0.0
% Calories from Fat: 26	Vegetable: 0.5
Fat (gm): 3.8	Fruit: 0.0
Saturated Fat (gm): 1.6	Bread: 1.0
Cholesterol (mg): 10.2	Meat: 0.5
Sodium (mg): 657	Fat: 0.5
Protein (gm): 7.4	
Carbohydrate (gm): 17	

Hawaiian Green Beans

1 8-ounce can crushed pineapple, in juice, undrained

3 tablespoons rice vinegar

1 tablespoon sugar

⅛ teaspoon freshly ground black pepper

1 tablespoon cornstarch

1 10-ounce package frozen French-cut green beans, thawed

1. Pour juice from pineapple into a saucepan. Set pineapple aside. Add vinegar, sugar, pepper, and cornstarch and mix well until cornstarch is completely dissolved.

2. Bring to a boil over medium-low heat and simmer 3 minutes or until thickened, stirring constantly. Stir in beans and pineapple and heat through.

SERVES 4 (½-cup servings)

Per Serving:
Calories: 58
% Calories from Fat: 2
Fat (gm): 0.2
Saturated Fat (gm): 0
Cholesterol (mg): 0
Sodium (mg): 10
Protein (gm): 1.2
Carbohydrate (gm): 14.6

Exchanges:
Milk: 0.0
Vegetable: 1.0
Fruit: 0.5
Bread: 0.0
Meat: 0.0
Fat: 0.0

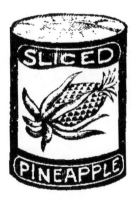

Honeyed Beets

This sweet-and-sour beet and onion side dish can be served hot or cold.

    1 16-ounce can sliced beets, undrained
    ¼ cup honey
    1 tablespoon cider vinegar
    1 tablespoon extra-virgin olive oil
    1 medium red onion, thinly sliced, separated into rings

1. Drain beets and pour all liquid into a saucepan. Add all remaining ingredients and bring to a boil over medium-low heat. Cool just until onions are crisp-tender, about 5 minutes.

2. Stir in beets and heat through if serving hot. If serving cold, refrigerate mixture in the cooking liquid. Drain before serving.

SERVES 4 (½-cup servings)

Per Serving:	*Exchanges:*
Calories: 141	Milk: 0.0
% Calories from Fat: 22	Vegetable: 2.0
Fat (gm): 3.6	Fruit: 1.0
Saturated Fat (gm): 0.5	Bread: 0.0
Cholesterol (mg): 0	Meat: 0.0
Sodium (mg): 313	Fat: 0.5
Protein (gm): 1.4	
Carbohydrate (gm): 28	

Herbed Scalloped Potatoes

This delicious potato dish can either be served as a side dish or as an entree.

3 15-ounce cans potatoes, drained, sliced

2 tablespoons flour

½ teaspoon salt

½ teaspoon freshly ground black pepper

¾ teaspoon dried oregano, crushed

¾ teaspoon dried basil, crushed

¾ cup shredded Parmesan cheese

1 onion, thinly sliced

1 12-ounce can evaporated skim milk

1. Preheat oven to 350°F. Spray a 9 x 13-in. baking dish with non-stick vegetable cooking spray. Layer bottom of dish with ⅓ of potatoes.

2. Combine flour, salt, pepper, oregano, and basil and mix well. Sprinkle ½ of flour mixture over potatoes. Then sprinkle ¼ cup of cheese over the top. Top cheese with ½ of the onion. Repeat with another layer of ½ of remaining potatoes, the remaining flour, another ¼ cup of cheese, and all remaining onions. Top with rest of potatoes and cheese.

3. Pour milk over top. Bake in preheated oven 1 hour or until bubbling and lightly browned.

SERVES 8 (⅔-cup servings)

Per Serving:
Calories: 188
% Calories from Fat: 16
Fat (gm): 3.3
Saturated Fat (gm): 1.9
Cholesterol (mg): 8.7
Sodium (mg): 773
Protein (gm): 9.8
Carbohydrate (gm): 30.3

Exchanges:
Milk: 0.5
Vegetable: 1.0
Fruit: 0.0
Bread: 1.0
Meat: 0.5
Fat: 0.5

Tuscan Potatoes

Although new potatoes are available stored, frozen, and canned all year around, nothing beats the taste and texture of the really "new" potatoes available only in the summer. While small red potatoes are often equated with new potatoes, any variety freshly dug that hasn't been stored can qualify in this category. My favorite recipe for new potatoes is this one that I learned at Badia a Coltibuono, Lorenzo de Medici's picturesque villa and cooking school in Tuscany. These tender garlic-and-rosemary-smothered potatoes are a perfect accompaniment for summer grilled menus. If you have any left over, serve them cold for a delicious and unusual potato salad.

1 16-ounce can new potatoes, drained, halved

1 tablespoon extra-virgin olive oil

6 garlic cloves, peeled

2 teaspoons dried rosemary, crushed

1. Preheat oven to 400°F. Combine all ingredients, except rosemary, in a 9 x 13-in. baking dish and mix until all potato pieces and garlic cloves are coated with oil. Sprinkle rosemary evenly over top. Bake in preheated oven about 45 minutes, stirring occasionally for even browning.

SERVES 3 (½-cup servings)

Per Serving:	*Exchanges:*
Calories: 142	Milk: 0.0
% Calories from Fat: 30	Vegetable: 0.0
Fat (gm): 5	Fruit: 0.0
Saturated Fat (gm): 0.7	Bread: 1.5
Cholesterol (mg): 0	Meat: 0.0
Sodium (mg): 395	Fat: 1.0
Protein (gm): 2.5	
Carbohydrate (gm): 23.1	

FIVE

Fish AND Seafood Entrees

*Most of my favorite pantry meals are in this section because of the
high quality and great variety available in canned fish and seafood.
Also, canned solid-pack white tuna can be substituted for
chicken in any of the recipes in the poultry section (Chapter 6).*

Tuna Tailgate Gumbo ☌ Tuna Tetrazzini ☌ Tuna Tamale Pie
Tuna Veracruzana ☌ Cheesy Smoked Tuna and Rice ☌ Crab
Cakes ☌ Cioppino ☌ Bouillabaisse ☌ Pantry Paella ☌ Teriyaki
Salmon and Vegetables on Brown Rice ☌ Salmon Mousse
Linguini with Clam Sauce ☌ Lobster à la Newburg

Tuna Tailgate Gumbo

For an easy-to-make and healthy meal that can be prepared right out of your pantry in less than twenty-five minutes and easily transported for a picnic or tailgate party, this gumbo is hard to beat. You can substitute either canned crab or shrimp for the tuna called for, but they are more expensive, and it takes three six-and-one-half-ounce cans of either crab or shrimp to equal the same volume as two six-ounce cans of tuna. If you want to inject a little more zing into your gumbo, add Tabasco sauce to taste. To complete the "pantry" menu for your next outing, pack a pan of cornbread to serve with the gumbo.

1 medium onion, chopped, *or* 1½ cups frozen chopped onions

2 cloves garlic, sliced

½ cup uncooked white rice

1 7-ounce jar roasted red sweet peppers, drained, chopped

3 cups shredded cabbage, *or* coleslaw mix

1 8-ounce can tomato sauce

1 8-ounce bottle clam juice

1 cup water

¾ teaspoon celery salt

½ teaspoon freshly ground black pepper

½ teaspoon dried thyme, crushed

¼ teaspoon red pepper flakes

2 bay leaves

1 12-ounce can solid-pack white tuna, in water, drained (*or* 2 6-ounce cans)

1 14½-ounce can chopped tomatoes, undrained

1 10-ounce package frozen sliced okra, thawed

Tabasco sauce, to taste (optional)

1. Combine onion and garlic in a heavy pot or soup kettle and cook, covered, over very low heat 5 minutes, adding a little water if necessary to prevent scorching.

2. Add all ingredients, except tuna, chopped tomatoes, and okra, and cook, covered, over medium-low heat 15 minutes or until most of the liquid has been absorbed and rice is completely cooked. Add remaining ingredients and cook, covered, until hot, about 2 minutes.

SERVES 8 (1¼-cup servings)

Per Serving:	*Exchanges:*
Calories: 164	Milk: 0.0
% Calories from Fat: 9	Vegetable: 2.0
Fat (gm): 1.6	Fruit: 0.0
Saturated Fat (gm): 0.4	Bread: 0.5
Cholesterol (mg): 17.9	Meat: 1.5
Sodium (mg): 664	Fat: 0.0
Protein (gm): 15.5	
Carbohydrate (gm): 23	

Tuna Tetrazzini

This is an easy and inexpensive dish that appeals to people of all ages. Canned chicken and turkey substitute well for the tuna called for in this recipe.

1 10¾-ounce can low-fat condensed cream of mushroom soup

1 10¾-ounce can low-fat condensed cream of chicken soup

3 tablespoons sherry

¼ teaspoon freshly ground black pepper

1 4-ounce jar sliced pimiento, drained

1 4-ounce can mushrooms, drained

1 12-ounce can white solid-pack tuna, in water, drained, flaked

8 ounces dry spaghetti, cooked *al dente* according to package directions, drained (4 cups cooked)

⅓ cups grated Parmesan cheese

1. Preheat oven to 400°F. Spray a 9 x 13-in. baking dish with non-stick vegetable cooking spray.

2. Combine soups, sherry, and pepper in a large bowl and mix well. Stir in pimientos, mushrooms, and tuna.

3. Add cooked spaghetti and mix well.

4. Spoon mixture into prepared dish and sprinkle cheese evenly over the top. Bake in preheated oven about 20 minutes or until bubbly.

SERVES 6 (1-cup servings)

Per Serving:
Calories: 301
% Calories from Fat: 15
Fat (gm): 4.9
Saturated Fat (gm): 1.6
Cholesterol (mg): 30.5
Sodium (mg): 623
Protein (gm): 23.9
Carbohydrate (gm): 37.1

Exchanges:
Milk: 0.0
Vegetable: 1.0
Fruit: 0.0
Bread: 2.0
Meat: 2.5
Fat: 0.0

Tuna Tamale Pie

For a vegetarian tamale pie, omit the tuna.

1 medium onion, chopped, *or* 1½ cups frozen chopped onions
1 garlic clove, pressed or minced
1 14½-ounce can chopped tomatoes, undrained
1 15-ounce can red kidney beans, drained
1 8-ounce can salt-free corn kernels, drained
¼ teaspoon salt
¼ teaspoon freshly ground black pepper
2 teaspoons chili powder
2 12-ounce cans white solid-pack tuna in water, drained, flaked
1 8½-ounce box cornbread mix
½ cup non-fat milk
1 egg, lightly beaten

1. Preheat oven to 350°F. Spray a 9 x 13-in. baking dish with non-stick vegetable cooking spray and set aside.

2. Cook onion and garlic in a heavy saucepan, covered, over low heat 10 minutes or until onion is translucent. Add tomatoes, beans, corn, salt, pepper, and chili powder and simmer, covered, 20 minutes. Add tuna and spoon mixture into the prepared baking dish.

3. Combine cornbread mix, milk, and egg in a bowl and mix well. Spoon mixture evenly over tuna mixture in the baking dish. Bake in preheated oven 20–25 minutes or until golden brown.

SERVES 8 (⅔-cup servings)

Per Serving:
Calories: 354
% Calories from Fat: 17
Fat (gm): 7.1
Saturated Fat (gm): 1.7
Cholesterol (mg): 62.6
Sodium (mg): 949
Protein (gm): 32.7
Carbohydrate (gm): 42.8

Exchanges:
Milk: 0.0
Vegetable: 1.0
Fruit: 0.0
Bread: 2.0
Meat: 3.5
Fat: 0.0

Tuna Veracruzana

This subtle, south-of-the-border flavor is typical of the state of Veracruz, Mexico, cooking style. It is usually made with fresh red snapper, but it is delicious with tuna. Try serving it over quick-cooking brown rice.

1 medium onion, chopped, *or* 1½ cups frozen chopped onions

2 14½-ounce cans chopped tomatoes, undrained

1 4-ounce can diced green chilies, undrained

2 teaspoons capers

1 tablespoon chopped fresh parsley (optional)

1 2-ounce jar slice pimientos

1 12-ounce can solid-pack white albacore tuna, packed in water, drained, flaked

1. Cook onion in a large, heavy saucepan, covered, over medium-low heat about 10 minutes or until soft and translucent, adding a little water if necessary to prevent scorching. Add tomatoes, chilies, capers, parsley, and pimientos and simmer 10 minutes. Add tuna and mix well.

SERVES 4 (1½ cup servings)

Per Serving:
Calories: 194
% Calories from Fat: 13
Fat (gm): 2.8
Saturated Fat (gm): 0.7
Cholesterol (mg): 35
Sodium (mg): 1034
Protein (gm): 25.7
Carbohydrate (gm): 17.4

Exchanges:
Milk: 0.0
Vegetable: 3.0
Fruit: 0.0
Bread: 0.0
Meat: 3.0
Fat: 0.0

Cheesy Smoked Tuna and Rice

To turn this simple, tasty treat into a one-dish meal, either serve it over your favorite vegetable or mix the vegetable into the tuna and rice. I like it best combined with baby peas.

1 12-ounce can evaporated skim milk

½ teaspoon dried dill weed, crushed

4 ounces (1 cup) fat-reduced sharp Cheddar cheese, grated

1½ cups instant rice, uncooked

2 6-ounce cans hickory-smoked tuna in water, undrained

2 tablespoons chopped fresh parsley (optional)

1. Combine milk and dill weed in a saucepan and bring to a boil over medium-low heat. Add cheese and cook, stirring constantly, until cheese is melted. Stir in rice, tuna, and (optional) parsley. Cover and remove from heat. Allow to stand 10 minutes or until all liquid is absorbed. Stir before serving.

SERVES 4 (1-cup servings)

Per Serving:	*Exchanges:*
Calories: 380	Milk: 0.5
% Calories from Fat: 12	Vegetable: 0.0
Fat (gm): 4.7	Fruit: 0.0
Saturated Fat (gm): 2.3	Bread: 2.0
Cholesterol (mg): 32.5	Meat: 4.0
Sodium (mg): 776	Fat: 0.0
Protein (gm): 39.4	
Carbohydrate (gm): 41.5	

Crab Cakes

⅓ cup non-fat mayonnaise

Pinch each: ground celery seed, ground ginger, and paprika

1 garlic clove, pressed or minced

2 teaspoons Worcestershire sauce

¼ teaspoon freshly ground black pepper

⅛ teaspoon ground celery seeds

⅛ teaspoon dry mustard

⅛ teaspoon red pepper flakes

1 cup soft breadcrumbs (2 slices bread)

2 6-ounce cans white crab meat, drained, rinsed

1. Combine all ingredients in a large bowl and mix well. Cover and refrigerate until well chilled. Form into 8 2-ounce patties and cook in a non-stick skillet over medium-low heat until brown on both sides.

SERVES 4 (2-patty servings)

Per Serving:	*Exchanges:*
Calories: 135	Milk: 0.0
% Calories from Fat: 17	Vegetable: 0.0
Fat (gm): 2.5	Fruit: 0.0
Saturated Fat (gm): 0.5	Bread: 0.5
Cholesterol (mg): 85.1	Meat: 2.0
Sodium (mg): 761	Fat: 0.0
Protein (gm): 16.2	
Carbohydrate (gm): 11	

Cioppino

The Italian fishermen who came to San Francisco during the great Gold Rush combined the local seafood and their native marinara sauce to create this fabulous, spicy stew.

1 26-ounce jar tomato and basil pasta sauce

1 8-ounce bottle clam juice

½ cup dry white wine

1 tablespoon lemon juice

2 tablespoons fresh parsley (optional)

1 6-ounce can white crab meat, drained, rinsed

1 6½-ounce can chopped clams, undrained

1 6-ounce can solid-pack white albacore tuna, packed in water, drained, flaked

1. Combine pasta sauce, clam juice, wine, lemon juice, and (optional) parsley and bring to a boil. Reduce heat to low and simmer 10 minutes. Add all seafood and heat through. Overcooking will toughen the seafood.

SERVES 6 (1-cup servings)

Per Serving:
Calories: 206
% Calories from Fat: 17
Fat (gm): 3.9
Saturated Fat (gm): 0.4
Cholesterol (mg): 59.4
Sodium (mg): 722
Protein (gm): 17.9
Carbohydrate (gm): 20.8

Exchanges:
Milk: 0.0
Vegetable: 4.0
Fruit: 0.0
Bread: 0.0
Meat: 2.0
Fat: 0.0

Bouillabaisse

This aromatic seafood stew is a staple of the fishermen on the southern coast of France around Marseilles. They serve it over crusty French bread, but I prefer to serve the bread on the side. For a bit fancier dish, substitute a can of lobster for the tuna. For a less expensive dish, substitute tuna for the crab.

1 medium onion, chopped, *or* 1½ cups frozen chopped onions

2 garlic cloves, pressed or minced

1 14½-ounce can chopped tomatoes, undrained

1 bay leaf

¼ teaspoon ground fennel seed

¼ teaspoon dried thyme, crushed

¼ teaspoon saffron

⅛ teaspoon freshly ground black pepper

2 8-ounce bottles clam juice

1 cup dry white wine

2 6½-ounce cans white crab meat, drained, rinsed

1 6½-ounce can chopped clams, undrained

1 6-ounce can solid-pack white tuna, packed in water

1. Combine onion and garlic in a heavy saucepan and cook, covered, over medium-low heat 10 minutes or until onion is soft and translucent. Add all other ingredients, except crab, clams, and tuna, and bring to a boil. Reduce heat to low and simmer, covered, 10 minutes. Add crab, clams, and tuna and mix well. Overcooking seafood will toughen it.

SERVES 6 (1⅓ cup servings)

Per Serving:	*Exchanges:*
Calories: 177	Milk: 0.0
% Calories from Fat: 14	Vegetable: 1.0
Fat (gm): 2.8	Fruit: 0.0
Saturated Fat (gm): 0.6	Bread: 0.0
Cholesterol (mg): 92.5	Meat: 3.0
Sodium (mg): 651	Fat: 0.0
Protein (gm): 23.2	
Carbohydrate (gm): 8.4	

Pantry Paella

This is the easiest recipe imaginable for this popular Spanish dish. For a more classic presentation, spoon the mixture into a large, flat serving dish and use the sliced pimientos to garnish the top instead of stirring them in at the end. For a less expensive version, you can substitute turmeric for the saffron, which will give it much the same shade of yellow. However, it is the saffron that gives paella its truly distinctive flavor, as well as the brilliant color.

1 tablespoon extra-virgin olive oil

1 medium onion, chopped, *or* 1, 12-ounce bag frozen chopped onions

2 garlic cloves, pressed or minced

2 cups uncooked white rice

1 5-ounce can extra-lean chunk ham

1 7-ounce jar roasted red sweet peppers, drained, cut into ½-in. strips

1 8-ounce can tomato sauce

1 14½-ounce can ready-cut tomatoes, undrained

½ teaspoon salt

½ teaspoon saffron

2 cups clam juice (2, 8-ounce bottles)

2 cups dry white wine

2 6½-ounce cans chopped clams

1 10-ounce can chunk white chicken, in water, undrained

1½ cups frozen peas, thawed

1 4-ounce jar sliced pimiento, undrained

1. Heat olive oil in a heavy pot with a tight-fitting lid. Add onion and garlic and cook over low heat, covered, 5 minutes. Add rice and ham and mix well. Add roasted pepper strips, tomato sauce, canned tomatoes, salt, saffron, clam juice, and wine.

2. Drain canned clams and add the juice from the cans to the mixture; set clams aside. Bring to a boil over medium heat. Reduce heat to low and simmer, covered, 20 minutes or until rice is tender.

3. Stir in reserved clams, chicken, peas, and pimiento. Remove from heat and allow to stand, covered, 5 more minutes.

SERVES 8 (1½-cup servings)

Per Serving:
Calories: 363
% Calories from Fat: 9
Fat (gm): 3.8
Saturated Fat (gm): 0.7
Cholesterol (mg): 5.3
Sodium (mg): 927
Protein (gm): 19.8
Carbohydrate (gm): 53.5

Exchanges:
Milk: 0.0
Vegetable: 2.0
Fruit: 0.0
Bread: 3.0
Meat: 2.0
Fat: 0.0

Teriyaki Salmon and Vegetables on Brown Rice

The flavor combination of teriyaki sauce and salmon is surprisingly good. If you have any leftovers, combine the salmon and vegetables with the rice and refrigerate for a delicious cold salad.

1¾ cups water

1 cup quick-cooking brown rice

⅓ cup low-sodium teriyaki sauce

1 tablespoon lemon juice

1 16-ounce bag stir-fry vegetables

1 14¾-ounce can salmon

1. Bring water to a boil in a saucepan with a tight-fitting lid. Stir in rice and return to a boil. Reduce heat to low and cook, covered, 5 minutes. Remove from heat and stir. Cover again and allow to stand at least 5 more minutes. Fluff with a fork before serving.

2. While the rice is cooking, pour teriyaki sauce and lemon juice into a wok or large skillet and bring to a boil. Add vegetables and cook, stirring constantly, over medium-high heat 2 minutes or until thawed. Add salmon and continue to cook 1 more minute.

3. To serve, spoon ⅔ cup rice onto each of 4 plates and top each serving with 1¼ cups of the salmon and vegetable mixture.

SERVES 4

Per Serving:
Calories: 370
% Calories from Fat: 18
Fat (gm): 7.4
Saturated Fat (gm): 1.8
Cholesterol (mg): 40.6
Sodium (mg): 934
Protein (gm): 27.6
Carbohydrate (gm): 46.3

Exchanges:
Milk: 0.0
Vegetable: 1.0
Fruit: 0.0
Bread: 2.5
Meat: 3.0
Fat: 0.0

Salmon Mousse

In most recipes calling for canned salmon you are told to discard the bones. I leave them in because they are enormously high in calcium and too soft to adversely affect the texture of the mousse. However, I do remove and discard the skin to lower the fat content. I like to serve this mousse with a sweet brown mustard or Dill Sauce (see page 18) and whole-grain rolls to help balance the percentage of calories from fat in the meal. You can also use this mousse as a sandwich spread or dip.

1 envelope unflavored gelatin
2 tablespoons cool water
¼ cup boiling water
½ cup fat-free mayonnaise
½ cup fat-free sour cream
⅛ teaspoon salt
½ teaspoon paprika
3 tablespoons lemon juice
1 14¾-ounce can red salmon, flaked, skin discarded

1. Spray a 3-quart mold with non-stick cooking spray and set aside.

2. In a small bowl, soften gelatin in cool water. Add boiling water and stir until completely dissolved.

3. In a large bowl, combine mayonnaise, sour cream, salt, paprika, lemon juice, and dissolved gelatin and mix well. Add salmon and again mix well. Spoon mixture into the prepared mold and refrigerate several hours or overnight before unmolding.

SERVES 6

Per Serving:	Exchanges:
Calories: 135	Milk: 0.0
% Calories from Fat: 33	Vegetable: 0.0
Fat (gm): 4.9	Fruit: 0.0
Saturated Fat (gm): 1.1	Bread: 0.5
Cholesterol (mg): 28.8	Meat: 2.0
Sodium (mg): 668	Fat: 0.0
Protein (gm): 15.8	
Carbohydrate (gm): 6.6	

Linguini with Clam Sauce

This fifteen-minute marvel has long been my favorite pantry meal. If you want to make it still lower in fat, just eliminate the oil and add the garlic to the undrained clams before heating them.

6 ounces dry linguini noodles (3 cups cooked)

1 tablespoon extra-virgin olive oil

1 garlic clove pressed or minced

1 6½-ounce can minced clams, undrained

¼ cups (2 ounces) shredded Parmesan cheese

1. Cook linguini according to package directions.

2. While pasta is cooking, heat olive oil and garlic in skillet just until garlic starts to sizzle. Add clams and all juice from can and heat through. Do not bring to boil because it will toughen clams.

3. To serve, spoon ½ of cooked pasta onto each plate or into each bowl. Top each serving with 3 tablespoons clam sauce and 2 tablespoons cheese. Serve immediately.

SERVES 2

Per Serving:
Calories: 546
% Calories from Fat: 25
Fat (gm): 14.6
Saturated Fat (gm): 3.8
Cholesterol (mg): 71.5
Sodium (mg): 349
Protein (gm): 40.3
Carbohydrate (gm): 61.1

Exchanges:
Milk: 0.0
Vegetable: 0.0
Fruit: 0.0
Bread: 4.0
Meat: 4.0
Fat: 1.0

Lobster à la Newburg

This French-sounding dish was actually created by a chef at Delmonico's in New York many years ago for a regular customer named Wenburg. When the gentleman and the restaurant had a falling out, the chef renamed the dish Newburg, which it is to this day. Even though the original recipe is far more complicated than this one, this is still a delicious and opulent dish. If you wish to make it more economically, just substitute solid-pack white tuna in water for the lobster. Serve the Newburg over rice or toast.

1 10¾-ounce can low-fat, condensed cream of mushroom soup
½ cup sherry
½ teaspoon paprika
⅛ teaspoon nutmeg
1 egg, lightly beaten
2 5-ounce cans lobster

1. Combine soup, sherry, paprika, and nutmeg in a saucepan and bring to a boil over medium-low heat. Add a little of the hot sauce to the egg and mix well. Stir egg mixture back into sauce. Add lobster and mix well. Remove from heat and serve immediately over rice or toast (not included in nutritional data).

SERVES 4 (¾-cup servings)

Per Serving:
Calories: 149
% Calories from Fat: 15
Fat (gm): 2.4
Saturated Fat (gm): 0.5
Cholesterol (mg): 105.8
Sodium (mg): 649
Protein (gm): 16.5
Carbohydrate (gm): 6.5

Exchanges:
Milk: 0.0
Vegetable: 0.0
Fruit: 0.0
Bread: 0.5
Meat: 2.0
Fat: 0.0

SIX

Poultry Entrees

Of all the canned poultry available, my favorite is the chunk white chicken packed in water, primarily because it is the most tender. However, if you are using the chicken in a sauce or soup, you may want to use a dark and light meat combination, which is less expensive. Also, if you have any leftover chicken or turkey in your refrigerator or freezer, you can certainly substitute it for the canned products and save even more money. Remember, too, that canned solid-packed white tuna can always be substituted for chicken in the following recipes.

Chicken Stew Provençal ❧ Chicken in Peachy Port Sauce on Spiced Couscous ❧ Chicken Linguini with Red Pepper Sauce ❧ Sweet-and-Sour Chicken on Jasmine Rice ❧ Curried Chicken and Rice ❧ Chicken and Broccoli Almondine ❧ Greek Chicken with Orzo Chicken Enchilada Casserole ❧ Chicken Tonnato Pasta ❧ Jambalaya

Chicken Stew Provençal

This flavorful stew is wonderful with crusty French bread and garlic-flavored mayonnaise. To make the garlic mayonnaise, just add a little fresh minced garlic or garlic paste and a teaspoon or two of extra-virgin olive oil to some fat-free or fat-reduced mayonnaise. Or make the cholesterol-free Light Aioli on page 20.

1 medium onion, chopped, *or* 1½ cups frozen chopped onions

3 garlic cloves, pressed or minced

1 28-ounce can chopped tomatoes, undrained

2 bay leaves

2 teaspoons dried thyme, crushed

½ teaspoon freshly ground black pepper

¼ teaspoon red pepper flakes

¼ cup Pernod (divided)

1 14½-ounce can fat-free, sodium-reduced chicken stock

1 15-ounce can new potatoes, drained

1 16-ounce bag frozen mixed vegetables

2 10-ounce cans chunk white chicken in water

1. Combine onions, garlic, undrained tomatoes, bay leaves, thyme, pepper, and red pepper flakes in a large pot or soup kettle and bring to a boil. Add 2 tablespoons of the Pernod and simmer 30 minutes. Add remaining Pernod and all other ingredients, except chicken, and cook 10 more minutes. Add chicken and mix well.

SERVES 8 (1½-cup servings)

Per Serving:	Exchanges:
Calories: 196	Milk: 0.0
% Calories from Fat: 7	Vegetable: 3.0
Fat (gm): 1.5	Fruit: 0.0
Saturated Fat (gm): 0.1	Bread: 0.5
Cholesterol (mg): 0	Meat: 2.0
Sodium (mg): 650	Fat: 0.0
Protein (gm): 22	
Carbohydrate (gm): 24.5	

Chicken in Peachy Port Sauce
on Spiced Couscous

This dish offers an interesting combination of flavors and textures. It is also good made with canned apricots or pears in place of the peaches and can be served over rice or any type of pasta if you don't have couscous.

Couscous

> 1 cup water
>
> ⅛ teaspoon freshly ground black pepper
>
> ⅛ teaspoon ground allspice
>
> 1 bay leaf
>
> ½ cup dry quick-cooking couscous

Chicken and Sauce

> 1 16-ounce can sliced peaches, packed in water, undrained
>
> ¼ cup port wine
>
> ¼ teaspoon salt
>
> ¼ teaspoon freshly ground black pepper
>
> ½ teaspoon dried oregano, crushed
>
> ⅛ teaspoon ground nutmeg
>
> 1 5-ounce can chunk white chicken in water, undrained

1. To make couscous, combine all ingredients, except dry couscous, in a saucepan and bring to a boil. Add couscous and mix well. Remove from heat and cover tightly. Allow to stand 5 minutes or until all liquid is absorbed.

2. Drain peaches and pour liquid into a blender or food processor. Add ½ of the peaches to blender, reserving remaining peaches to add later. Add the port and all remaining ingredients, except the chicken, to blender and puree.

3. Pour pureed mixture into a saucepan. Add reserved peaches and bring to a boil. Reduce heat to medium-low and simmer, uncovered, 10 minutes, stirring frequently. Add chicken and mix well. Return to simmer and immediately remove from heat.

4. To serve, spoon couscous onto serving plate and top with chicken mixture; or spoon ¾ cup couscous onto individual plates and top each serving with 1 cup of the chicken mixture.

SERVES 2

Per Serving:
Calories: 358
% Calories from Fat: 4
Fat (gm): 1.6
Saturated Fat (gm): 0.1
Cholesterol (mg): 0
Sodium (mg): 533
Protein (gm): 24.3
Carbohydrate (gm): 56.2

Exchanges:
Milk: 0.0
Vegetable: 0.0
Fruit: 1.0
Bread: 2.5
Meat: 2.0
Fat: 0.0

Chicken Linguini with Red Pepper Sauce

This is a true cupboard combination! To make it even more delicious, use freshly grated Parmesan or Romano cheese.

12 ounces dry linguini (6 cups cooked)

1 26-ounce jar spicy fat-free pasta sauce

¾ teaspoon dried rosemary, crushed

1 10-ounce can chunk white chicken in water

¾ cup shredded Parmesan cheese (optional)

1. Cook linguini *al dente* according to package directions.

2. While pasta is cooking, combine pasta sauce and rosemary in a saucepan and cook over medium-low heat until it comes to boil. Reduce heat to low and simmer 5 minutes. Stir in chicken and remove from heat.

3. To serve, pour ¾ cup of sauce over 1½ cups of pasta on each of 4 plates. Top each serving with 3 tablespoons Parmesan cheese, if desired.

SERVES 4

Per Serving:
Calories: 508
% Calories from Fat: 7
Fat (gm): 4
Saturated Fat (gm): 0.2
Cholesterol (mg): 18.8
Sodium (mg): 386
Protein (gm): 32
Carbohydrate (gm): 84.8

Exchanges:
Milk: 0.0
Vegetable: 3.0
Fruit: 0.0
Bread: 4.0
Meat: 2.5
Fat: 0.0

Sweet-and-Sour Chicken on Jasmine Rice

If you prefer, you can combine the rice and chicken mixture. This works particularly well for a buffet party because you only need to put one dish on the table. I like to serve this dish with pea pods, broccoli florets, or a brightly colored combination of stir-fried vegetables.

2 cups water

1 cup uncooked jasmine rice, *or* any regular white rice

1 8-ounce can pineapple chunks, in juice, undrained

1½ tablespoons cornstarch

¼ teaspoon salt

1½ teaspoons sugar

2 tablespoons cider vinegar

1½ teaspoons sodium-reduced soy sauce

1 small onion, thinly sliced

1 8-ounce can sliced water chestnuts, drained

1 4-ounce can sliced mushrooms, drained

1 10-ounce can chunk white chicken in water, undrained

1. Combine water and rice in a saucepan with a tight-fitting lid. Bring to a boil. Reduce heat to low and simmer, covered, about 15 minutes or until all liquid is absorbed. Fluff with a fork before serving.

2. Pour juice from pineapple into a saucepan, reserving chunks to add later. Stir in cornstarch until completely dissolved. Add salt, sugar, vinegar, and soy sauce and cook over medium heat, stirring constantly, until thickened. Add pineapple chunks, onion, water chestnuts, and mushrooms and cook until onion is crisp-tender. Stir in chicken.

3. To serve, spoon ¾ cup of rice onto each of 4 plates, and spoon 1 cup of the chicken mixture over each serving.

SERVES 4

Per Serving:	*Exchanges:*
Calories: 345	Milk: 0.0
% Calories from Fat: 4	Vegetable: 1.0
Fat (gm): 1.5	Fruit: 0.5
Saturated Fat (gm): 0.1	Bread: 3.0
Cholesterol (mg): 0	Meat: 2.0
Sodium (mg): 582	Fat: 0.0
Protein (gm): 22.2	
Carbohydrate (gm): 63	

Curried Chicken and Rice

By omitting the rice, this delicious, mildly flavored curried chicken sauce can double as a soup, and it is also good cold. When serving it as a cold soup, I puree it in a blender with three tablespoons of mango chutney and serve it with cinnamon rice cakes.

1 10¾-ounce can low-fat condensed cream of chicken soup

1 10¾-ounce can low-fat condensed cream of mushroom soup

1 12-ounce can evaporated skim milk

1 teaspoon curry powder

½ teaspoon turmeric

¼ teaspoon ground ginger

1 10-ounce can chunk white chicken in water

4 cups cooked rice

1. Combine chicken soup and mushroom soup in a blender and puree.

2. Combine pureed soups and all remaining ingredients, except chicken and rice, in a saucepan and slowly bring to a simmer. Add chicken and rice, mix well, and heat through.

3. For each serving, spoon 1⅓ cups of mixture onto each plate. If making ahead of time, reheat to desired temperature but do not boil.

SERVES 6

Per Serving:
Calories: 152
% Calories from Fat: 11
Fat (gm): 1.8
Saturated Fat (gm): 0.1
Cholesterol (mg): 4
Sodium (mg): 441
Protein (gm): 16.8
Carbohydrate (gm): 17.5

Exchanges:
Milk: 0.0
Vegetable: 0.0
Fruit: 0.0
Bread: 1.0
Meat: 1.5
Fat: 0.2

Chicken and Broccoli Almondine

This is also good served with pasta in place of the rice.

2 tablespoons chopped raw almonds

1 medium onion, chopped, *or* 1½ cups frozen chopped onions

1 16-ounce package frozen broccoli florets, thawed

1 10¾-ounce can low-fat condensed cream of mushroom soup

1 4-ounce can sliced mushrooms

½ teaspoon freshly ground black pepper

⅛ teaspoon red pepper flakes

4 ounces fat-reduced sharp Cheddar cheese, grated (1 cup)

1 10-ounce can white chunk chicken in water

3 cups cooked brown rice

1. Put almonds in a skillet and cook over medium heat, stirring frequently, until well toasted. Set aside.

2. Cook onion in a large, heavy pan, covered, over medium-low heat 10 minutes or until onion is translucent, adding a little water if necessary to prevent scorching. Uncover and add broccoli. Continue to cook, stirring frequently, until broccoli is hot. Add mushroom soup, mushrooms, pepper, and red pepper flakes and mix well. Stir in cheese and continue to cook, stirring frequently, until cheese is melted. Stir in chicken and rice. Top each serving with a teaspoon of toasted almonds.

SERVES 6 (1½-cup servings)

Per Serving:	*Exchanges:*
Calories: 280	Milk: 0.0
% Calories from Fat: 20	Vegetable: 1.5
Fat (gm): 6.3	Fruit: 0.0
Saturated Fat (gm): 1.7	Bread: 1.5
Cholesterol (mg): 11.2	Meat: 2.5
Sodium (mg): 633	Fat: 0.0
Protein (gm): 22	
Carbohydrate (gm): 36.2	

Greek Chicken with Orzo

When making this dish, it is easier to cut the dried tomatoes into strips using scissors rather than a knife. It is great served hot as a one-dish meal for buffet entertaining, and it is also good served cold or at room temperature as a pasta salad.

1 tablespoon extra-virgin olive oil

3 cloves garlic, pressed or minced

1 medium onion, thinly sliced

1 7-ounce jar roasted red sweet peppers, cut into thin strips

1 cup (2 ounces) dried tomatoes, cut into thin strips

1 cup dry white wine

1 teaspoon ground cinnamon

½ teaspoon dried oregano, crushed

2 teaspoons honey

¼ teaspoon salt

¼ teaspoon freshly ground black pepper

1 10-ounce can chunk chicken in water, undrained

8 ounces dry orzo pasta (4 cups cooked)

1. Heat oil and garlic in a large skillet over medium heat just until it sizzles. Add onion and cook, stirring frequently, until onion is translucent. Add remaining ingredients, except chicken and orzo, and bring to a boil. Reduce heat and simmer, stirring frequently, for 15 minutes.

2. While the sauce is cooking, cook orzo according to package directions and drain thoroughly. Stir chicken and drained orzo into the sauce and heat through.

SERVES 4 (1¼-cup servings)

Per Serving: Exchanges:
Calories: 444   Milk: 0.0
% Calories from Fat: 12   Vegetable: 2.0
Fat (gm): 6   Fruit: 0.0
Saturated Fat (gm): 0.7   Bread: 3.5
Cholesterol (mg): 0   Meat: 2.5
Sodium (mg): 676   Fat: 0.0
Protein (gm): 27.5
Carbohydrate (gm): 63.7

Chicken Enchilada Casserole

This casserole can be made ahead of time and then baked just before you plan to serve it. If you put it in the oven directly from the refrigerator, allow a few more minutes baking time.

1 10¾-ounce can low-fat condensed cream of chicken soup

½ cup non-fat milk

½ cup fat-free sour cream

1 medium onion, finely chopped, *or* 1½ cups frozen chopped onions

1 4-ounce can diced green chilies

12 corn tortillas, shredded

2 10-ounce cans chunk white chicken in water, flaked

2 ounces fat-reduced sharp Cheddar cheese, grated (½ cup)

1. Preheat oven to 350°F. Spray a 9 x 13-in. baking pan with non-stick vegetable cooking spray.

2. Combine soup, milk, sour cream, onion, and diced chilies in a bowl and mix well.

3. Spread one-half of shredded tortillas evenly in the bottom of prepared pan. Top tortillas with one-half of the chicken. Top chicken with one-half of the soup mixture. Repeat layers and top with cheese. Bake 30 minutes or until hot and bubbly.

SERVES 6

Per Serving:
Calories: 296
% Calories from Fat: 13
Fat (gm): 4.5
Saturated Fat (gm): 0.9
Cholesterol (mg): 6.5
Sodium (mg): 895
Protein (gm): 30.6
Carbohydrate (gm): 36.1

Exchanges:
Milk: 0.0
Vegetable: 1.0
Fruit: 0.0
Bread: 2.0
Meat: 2.5
Fat: 0.0

Chicken Tonnato Pasta

Tonnato sauce is usually served over veal, but it is delicious over chicken. This dish can be served as an appetizer or an entree. You can also serve it over rice, or use the tonnato sauce as a dip with toast, chips, or crackers.

½ cup fat-free mayonnaise

1 6-ounce can water-packed tuna

1 tablespoon anchovy paste

1 tablespoon lemon juice

Dash cayenne pepper

1 tablespoon extra-virgin olive oil

12 ounces dry pasta shells, cooked according to package directions
(6 cups cooked), drained

2 10-ounce cans chunk white chicken in water, drained

1. Combine all ingredients, except olive oil, chicken, and pasta, in a blender or food processor and blend until smooth. Slowly add oil while blender is running.

2. To serve, put 1½ cups of pasta on each of 4 plates. You can either top each serving with ½ cup of chicken and ⅓ cup of sauce, or mix chicken and sauce together with the pasta.

SERVES 4

Per Serving:
Calories: 612
% Calories from Fat: 12
Fat (gm): 8.5
Saturated Fat (gm): 1.2
Cholesterol (mg): 27
Sodium (mg): 1065
Protein (gm): 58.2
Carbohydrate (gm): 76.2

Exchanges:
Milk: 0.0
Vegetable: 0.0
Fruit: 0.0
Bread: 5.0
Meat: 7.0
Fat: 0.0

Jambalaya

This is a Creole dish that varies widely from one southern cook to another, but they all include rice, onions, tomatoes, peppers, and ham. In fact, the name, jambalaya, comes from the French word for ham, jambon. *However, since there is more chicken than ham in this recipe, I decided to put it in the poultry section.*

1 medium onion, chopped, *or* 1½ cups frozen chopped onions

1 garlic clove, pressed or minced

1 7-ounce jar roasted red sweet peppers, drained, chopped

1 8-ounce can low-sodium tomato sauce

2 bay leaves

½ teaspoon freshly ground black pepper

½ teaspoon paprika

¼ teaspoon cayenne pepper

½ teaspoon dried oregano, crushed

½ teaspoon dried thyme, crushed

½ teaspoon dried basil, crushed

1 14½-ounce can fat-free, sodium-reduced chicken stock

1 5-ounce can extra-lean chunk ham

1 cup uncooked white rice

1 10-ounce can chunk white chicken in water

Tabasco sauce, to taste

1. Combine garlic and onion in a heavy pan and cook, covered, over medium-low heat 10 minutes or until onion is translucent, adding a little water if necessary to prevent scorching. Add all ingredients, except rice and chicken, and bring to a boil. Add rice and cook, covered, over low heat 20 minutes or until rice is tender. Stir in chicken and serve.

SERVES 4 (1½-cup servings)

Per Serving:
Calories: 373
% Calories from Fat: 8
Fat (gm): 3.4
Saturated Fat (gm): 0.7
Cholesterol (mg): 10.6
Sodium (mg): 829
Protein (gm): 32.5
Carbohydrate (gm): 53.8

Exchanges:
Milk: 0.0
Vegetable: 2.0
Fruit: 0.0
Bread: 2.5
Meat: 3.0
Fat: 0.0

SEVEN

Meat Dishes

In this section, I always call for five-ounce cans of ham rather than the larger canned hams because I routinely use the entire contents of all cans in each recipe. However, if you want to increase the volume of these recipes, you may find that buying a one-pound canned ham and chopping it up is more economical. The reason I always use canned beef in gravy is because that is the only way it comes. I don't particularly like the flavor, so I always drain, rinse, and shred the beef to better absorb the taste of the other ingredients in the recipe.

Beef and Vegetable Stew ❻ Beef Barbecue Cups
Beef Stroganoff ❻ Southwestern Beef and Bean
Lasagna ❻ Macronade ❻ Beef and Tomato Curry
Speedy Sukiyaki ❻ Red Flannel Hash ❻ Ham in
Orange Sauce on Wild Rice ❻ Ham and Pineapple
with Spiced Couscous ❻ Alsatian Ham and
Sauerkraut with New Potatoes

Beef and Vegetable Stew

1 medium onion, chopped, *or* 12-ounce bag frozen chopped onions

1 clove garlic, pressed or minced

1 8-ounce can sliced mushrooms, drained

½ teaspoon dried thyme, crushed

½ teaspoon dried dill weed, crushed

½ teaspoon summer savory, crushed

1 bay leaf

½ teaspoon freshly ground black pepper

1 12-ounce can roast beef in gravy, drained, rinsed, and shredded

2 cups dry red wine

1½ cups water

1 16-ounce can onions, drained

1 cup frozen baby carrots, *or* 16-ounce can whole carrots, drained

12 frozen new potatoes, *or* 2, 15-ounce cans new potatoes, drained

2 cups frozen peas, *or* 2 8½-ounce cans peas, drained

3 tablespoons all-purpose flour

¼ cup water

1. Combine onions, garlic, and mushrooms in a large pot or soup kettle and cook, covered, over medium-low heat 5 minutes. Add all remaining ingredients, except peas, flour, and water, and simmer, covered, 30 minutes. Add peas and cook 10 more minutes.

2. Combine flour and water and stir until flour is completely dissolved. Add mixture to the stew and cook, stirring constantly, until slightly thickened.

SERVES 6 (1¾-cup servings)

Per Serving:	*Exchanges:*
Calories: 322	Milk: 0.0
% Calories from Fat: 5	Vegetable: 1.5
Fat (gm): 1.7	Fruit: 0.0
Saturated Fat (gm): 0.6	Bread: 3.0
Cholesterol (mg): 23.6	Meat: 1.5
Sodium (mg): 633	Fat: 0.0
Protein (gm): 17.2	
Carbohydrate (gm): 49.4	

Beef Barbecue Cups

These tasty little treats are also good served at room temperature and can be packed for picnics or school lunches.

1 small onion, chopped, *or* 1 cup frozen chopped onions

¼ cup barbecue sauce

1 tablespoon, packed, dark brown sugar

1 9¾-ounce can roast beef in gravy, drained, rinsed, and shredded

1 7½-ounce can refrigerated biscuits

1¾ ounces (scant ½ cup) fat-reduced sharp Cheddar cheese, grated

1. Preheat oven to 400°F. Spray 10 of the 12 muffin cups in standard-size muffin tin with no-stick vegetable cooking spray.

2. Cook onions in a heavy pan, covered, over low heat 10 minutes or until translucent, adding a little water if necessary to prevent scorching. Stir in barbecue sauce, brown sugar, and shredded beef.

3. Place a biscuit in each sprayed muffin cup. Make a well in the center of each biscuit and fill with beef mixture. Bake in preheated oven about 10 minutes or until biscuits are golden brown. Remove from oven and sprinkle the tops with cheese.

SERVES 5 (2-biscuit servings)

Per Serving:	*Exchanges:*
Calories: 249	Milk: 0.0
% Calories from Fat: 32	Vegetable: 0.0
Fat (gm): 8.9	Fruit: 0.0
Saturated Fat (gm): 2.9	Bread: 1.5
Cholesterol (mg): 33.6	Meat: 1.5
Sodium (mg): 1014	Fat: 1.5
Protein (gm): 16.3	
Carbohydrate (gm): 26.6	

Beef Stroganoff

You can make this dish ahead of time, combine the noodles and meat mixture, and reheat it just before serving. You can also replace the beef with chicken if you prefer.

8 ounces dry noodles (4 cups cooked)

1 1.37-ounce package Chicken Dijon Sauce Blend

1 cup non-fat milk

½ cup non-fat sour cream

1 9¾-ounce can roast beef with gravy, drained, rinsed, and shredded

1. Cook noodles according to package directions. While noodles are cooking, combine sauce mix and milk in a saucepan and bring to a boil over medium-low heat, stirring constantly. Reduce heat to low and simmer 10 minutes or until thickened. Stir in sour cream and shredded beef and heat through. Do not allow to boil.

2. Place 1 cup cooked noodles on each of 4 plates, and top each serving with ½ cup of beef mixture.

SERVES 4

Per Serving:	*Exchanges:*
Calories: 366	Milk: 0.0
% Calories from Fat: 10	Vegetable: 0.0
Fat (gm): 4.1	Fruit: 0.0
Saturated Fat (gm): 1.5	Bread: 3.0
Cholesterol (mg): 39.3	Meat: 2.5
Sodium (mg): 866	Fat: 0.0
Protein (gm): 25.5	
Carbohydrate (gm): 56.5	

Southwestern Beef and Bean Lasagna

This recipe is a fabulous example of combining both the ingredients and methods of two entirely different cultural cuisines to create a delightful new dish.

1 medium onion, chopped, *or* 1½ cups frozen chopped onions

1 clove garlic, pressed or minced

4 cups low-sodium tomato sauce

1 4-ounce can diced green chilies

¼ teaspoon red pepper flakes

½ teaspoon ground cumin

1 teaspoon dried oregano, crushed

2 teaspoons chili powder

1 12-ounce can roast beef in gravy, drained, rinsed, and shredded

1 16-ounce can pinto beans, drained

8 ounces fat-free cottage cheese

6 ounces (1½ cups) fat-reduced reduced sharp Cheddar cheese, grated (divided)

1 egg white

¼ cup chopped fresh cilantro leaves (optional)

½ teaspoon freshly ground black pepper

8 ounces dry no-boil lasagna noodles

1 cup water

1. Combine onions and garlic and cook in a large skillet, covered, about 10 minutes or until onions are translucent. Add tomato sauce, green chilies, red pepper flakes, cumin, oregano, and chili powder and bring to a boil. Reduce heat to low and simmer, uncovered, 20 minutes.

2. Combine beef and beans, mix well, and set aside. Preheat oven to 350°F. Spray a 9 x 13-in. baking pan with non-stick vegetable cooking spray.

3. Combine cottage cheese, ½ cup of the Cheddar cheese, egg white, (optional) cilantro, and pepper in bowl and mix well.

4. To assemble, cover bottom of the prepared pan with ¾ cup of the tomato sauce mixture. Place a layer of noodles over sauce. Spread noodles with ½ of the beef mixture and then place another layer of noodles on top of beef. Spread cheese mixture over noodles and top with remaining beef mixture. Top beef

with remaining noodles and pour remaining tomato sauce evenly over them. Sprinkle remaining 1 cup of Cheddar cheese over the top.

5. Pour water around the edges and cover tightly with foil. Bake 1 hour and 15 minutes or until pasta is tender. Allow to cool 10 minutes before cutting.

SERVES 8

Per Serving:
Calories: 292
% Calories from Fat: 32
Fat (gm): 12.7
Saturated Fat (gm): 2
Cholesterol (mg): 35.2
Sodium (mg): 1064
Protein (gm): 23.2
Carbohydrate (gm): 38.5

Exchanges:
Milk: 0.0
Vegetable: 2.5
Fruit: 0.0
Bread: 1.5
Meat: 1.5
Fat: 1.0

Macronade

This hearty meat and pasta dish is famous in the region of Sete in the south of France. They usually serve it over rigatoni for a party, appropriately named Soirée Macronade.

1 medium onion, chopped, *or* 1½ cups frozen chopped onions

3 cloves garlic, pressed or minced

1 6-ounce can tomato paste

1 8-ounce can tomato paste

1 14½-ounce can chopped tomatoes, undrained

1 tablespoon sugar

1 9¾-ounce can roast beef in gravy, drained, rinsed, and shredded

1 5-ounce can extra-lean chunk ham

¾ cup dry red wine

¼ teaspoon freshly ground black pepper

⅛ teaspoon red pepper flakes

16 ounces dry rigatoni (8 cups cooked)

1. Combine onion and garlic in a heavy pot and cook, covered, over medium-low heat 10 minutes or until onions are translucent. Add tomato paste, tomato sauce, undrained chopped tomatoes, and sugar and bring to a boil. Reduce heat to low and simmer, covered, 1 hour, stirring occasionally. Add all remaining ingredients, except rigatoni, and continue to cook, covered, 30 more minutes.

2. Cook rigatoni *al dente* according to package directions and drain thoroughly. To serve, spoon 1½ cups rigatoni onto each of 6 plates, and top each serving with 1 cup of sauce.

SERVES 6

Per Serving:	*Exchanges:*
Calories: 468	Milk: 0.0
% Calories from Fat: 8	Vegetable: 2.0
Fat (gm): 4	Fruit: 0.0
Saturated Fat (gm): 1.2	Bread: 4.5
Cholesterol (mg): 30.7	Meat: 1.5
Sodium (mg): 980	Fat: 0.0
Protein (gm): 26.4	
Carbohydrate (gm): 76.8	

Beef and Tomato Curry

This hearty curry is good served over rice or Asian noodles. Serve chutney and other curry condiments such as peanuts and diced pineapple on the side.

1 medium onion, chopped, *or* 1½ cups frozen chopped onions

1 garlic clove, pressed or minced

1 9¾-ounce can roast beef in gravy, drained, rinsed, and shredded

1 14½-ounce can chopped tomatoes, undrained

1 8-ounce can tomato sauce

½ cup water

1 tablespoon honey

¼ cup raisins

2 teaspoons curry powder

¼ teaspoon ground cinnamon

¼ teaspoon ground allspice

¼ teaspoon ground ginger

¼ teaspoon freshly ground black pepper

1. Combine onion and garlic in a heavy saucepan and cook, covered, over medium-low heat 10 minutes or until onion is translucent, adding a little water if necessary to prevent scorching. Add all other ingredients and simmer 10 minutes.

SERVES 4 (1¼-cup servings)

Per Serving:	*Exchanges:*
Calories: 180	Milk: 0.0
% Calories from Fat: 10	Vegetable: 2.5
Fat (gm): 2.2	Fruit: 0.5
Saturated Fat (gm): 0.8	Bread: 0.0
Cholesterol (mg): 35.4	Meat: 1.5
Sodium (mg): 921	Fat: 0.0
Protein (gm): 16.1	
Carbohydrate (gm): 27.3	

Speedy Sukiyaki

Start cooking the rice about ten minutes ahead of time so that it will be ready to serve when the dish is finished. This dish is also good if the rice is replaced with soba noodles tossed with a teaspoon or two of dark sesame oil. If you have any sukiyaki left over, refrigerate it to serve as a chilled salad.

¼ cup sodium-reduced soy sauce

½ cup mirin (sweet sake)

¼ cup water

1 9¾-ounce can roast beef in gravy, drained, rinsed, and shredded

1 medium onion, thinly sliced

1 16-ounce package frozen spinach leaves, unthawed

1 10½-ounce package extra-firm tofu, cubed

4 cups cooked rice

1. Combine soy sauce, mirin, and water in bowl and mix well. Add shredded beef and set aside. (If you are not in a hurry, allow meat to marinate 1 hour.)

2. In large skillet, over medium heat, combine onion and spinach and cook, stirring constantly, until spinach is completely thawed. Add beef mixture with marinade and cook 1 more minute. Carefully stir in tofu cubes and cook 1 more minute or until tofu is thoroughly heated. Serve immediately over cooked rice.

SERVES 4 (1¾-cups servings)

Per Serving:	*Exchanges:*
Calories: 479	Milk: 0.0
% Calories from Fat: 34	Vegetable: 2.0
Fat (gm): 23.6	Fruit: 0.0
Saturated Fat (gm): 1.9	Bread: 3.0
Cholesterol (mg): 45.2	Meat: 3.0
Sodium (mg): 1118	Fat: 1.0
Protein (gm): 34.7	
Carbohydrate (gm): 63.2	

Red Flannel Hash

This hearty New England dish makes good use of leftover corned beef and vegetables. Although every recipe I have ever seen for this hash uses only beets and potatoes with the corned beef, I have occasionally added other leftover vegetables such as cooked carrots, parsnips, and cabbage and it was wonderful. You can also achieve the same result by combining all the canned ingredients for a great and satisfying last-minute meal.

1 tablespoon canola oil

1 medium onion, chopped, *or* 1½ cups frozen chopped onions

1 tablespoon imitation bacon chips

1 16-ounce can julienne beets, drained

1 16-ounce can new potatoes, drained and chopped

1 12-ounce can lean corned beef, crumbled

3 tablespoons light sour cream

¼ teaspoon freshly ground black pepper

2 tablespoons chopped fresh parsley (optional)

1. Heat oil in a large non-stick skillet. Add onion and bacon chips and cook, uncovered, over medium heat until onions are soft and browned.

2. Combine cooked onions and all remaining ingredients in a large bowl and mix well. Spoon mixture back into the skillet and press down firmly. Cook over medium-low heat about 20 minutes, stirring frequently for even browning.

SERVES 6 (½-cup servings)

Per Serving:	*Exchanges:*
Calories: 237	Milk: 0.0
% Calories from Fat: 38	Vegetable: 1.0
Fat (gm): 10.3	Fruit: 0.0
Saturated Fat (gm): 3.3	Bread: 1.0
Cholesterol (mg): 52.4	Meat: 2.0
Sodium (mg): 928	Fat: 0.5
Protein (gm): 17.8	
Carbohydrate (gm): 20	

Ham in Orange Sauce on Wild Rice

If you are really in a hurry and don't want to wait forty-five minutes for the wild rice to cook, use quick-cooking brown rice instead. It only takes ten minutes to cook and it is less expensive!

1 5-ounce box instant wild rice

1 cup water

1 tablespoon cornstarch

⅓ cup frozen orange juice concentrate, undiluted

1½ tablespoons light brown sugar

½ teaspoon ground cinnamon

⅛ teaspoon ground clove

¼ teaspoon red pepper flakes

2 5-ounce cans extra-lean ham, chopped

1. Prepare wild rice according to package directions. Leave covered while you make the ham mixture.

2. Combine water and cornstarch in a saucepan and stir until cornstarch is completely dissolved. Add all remaining ingredients, except ham and rice, and mix well. Cook over medium-low heat, stirring frequently, until thickened. Add ham and heat through.

3. To serve, spoon ⅔ cup of rice onto each of 4 plates and top each serving with ½ cup of ham mixture.

SERVES 4

Per Serving:
Calories: 297
% Calories from Fat: 12
Fat (gm): 3.9
Saturated Fat (gm): 1.2
Cholesterol (mg): 21.3
Sodium (mg): 823
Protein (gm): 20.1
Carbohydrate (gm): 44.4

Exchanges:
Milk: 0.0
Vegetable: 0.0
Fruit: 0.5
Bread: 2.0
Meat: 2.0
Fat: 0.0

Ham and Pineapple with Spiced Couscous

This is a wonderful holiday recipe, perfect for buffet parties. It is equally good served hot or chilled and served cold as a couscous salad.

1 20-ounce can crushed pineapple in juice, undrained

1 cup water

½ teaspoon ground cinnamon

¼ teaspoon salt

¼ teaspoon ground allspice

⅛ teaspoon ground clove

1 10-ounce box dry couscous

2 5-ounce cans extra-lean chunk ham, drained and flaked

1. Drain pineapple thoroughly and pour all juice from the can into a saucepan, reserving pineapple to add later. Add water, cinnamon, salt, allspice, and clove and bring to a boil.

2. Add couscous and mix well. Remove from heat and cover. Allow to stand 5 minutes or until all liquid has been absorbed. Stir in drained pineapple and ham. Serve hot or cold.

SERVES 5 (1⅓-cup servings)

Per Serving:	Exchanges:
Calories: 359	Milk: 0.0
% Calories from Fat: 8	Vegetable: 0.0
Fat (gm): 3.2	Fruit: 1.5
Saturated Fat (gm): 1	Bread: 2.5
Cholesterol (mg): 17	Meat: 2.0
Sodium (mg): 758	Fat: 0.0
Protein (gm): 19.7	
Carbohydrate (gm): 62.1	

Alsatian Ham and Sauerkraut
with New Potatoes

In the Alsace region of northeastern France, sauerkraut cooked with wine and juniper berries and served with either sausage or ham and potatoes is a very popular dish. For a variation and to reduce the amount of sodium per serving, serve only ¼ cup of ham and sauerkraut over large baked potatoes.

1 16-ounce can sauerkraut, rinsed and drained

1 cup white wine

2 teaspoons juniper berries

1 5-ounce can extra-lean chunk ham, flaked

1 15-ounce can new potatoes, drained

1. Combine drained sauerkraut, wine, and juniper berries in a saucepan and bring to a boil. Reduce heat to low and simmer, covered, 15 minutes. Add ham and potatoes and continue to cook, covered, 5 more minutes.

2. To serve, divide potatoes onto 4 plates and spoon ½ cup of ham and sauerkraut onto each serving.

SERVES 4

Per Serving:	*Exchanges:*
Calories: 174	Milk: 0.0
% Calories from Fat: 11	Vegetable: 1.0
Fat (gm): 2.1	Fruit: 0.0
Saturated Fat (gm): 0.7	Bread: 1.0
Cholesterol (mg): 10.6	Meat: 1.0
Sodium (mg): 1431	Fat: 0.0
Protein (gm): 10.1	
Carbohydrate (gm): 20	

EIGHT

Baked Goods, Breakfast, AND Such

Even though there are many light and excellent prepared mixes available, there are still a few of my favorite pantry recipes that I'll never give up, such as Oatmeal Pancakes and Rye and Raisin Cereal. I really don't like the taste or texture of packaged croutons and breadcrumbs, and it's so easy and inexpensive to make your own. For anyone who practically faints at the idea of baking bread, the Fast Focaccia is your kind of recipe!

Croutons

Packaged croutons are on my list of unacceptable convenience products. They taste terrible no matter how fresh they are and cost a lot more than making your own.

    4 slices bread, cut into ½-in. cubes

1. Preheat oven to 300°F. Place bread cubes in a flat baking pan, and bake about 25 minutes or until golden brown, turning several times for even browning. (Makes 2 cups.)

SERVES 8 (¼-cup servings)

Per Serving:	*Exchanges:*
Calories: 34	Milk: 0.0
% Calories from Fat: 12	Vegetable: 0.0
Fat (gm): 0.5	Fruit: 0.0
Saturated Fat (gm): 0.1	Bread: 0.5
Cholesterol (mg): 0	Meat: 0.0
Sodium (mg): 68	Fat: 0.0
Protein (gm): 1.1	
Carbohydrate (gm): 6.2	

Garlic Croutons

You can lower the fat content of these croutons by reducing the amount of olive oil used in the skillet. However, since you will be using the croutons primarily as a topping for relatively low-fat salads and the like, the percentage of calories from fat will probably be reduced by the rest of the meal.

    2 tablespoons extra-virgin olive oil
    1 garlic clove, pressed or minced
    4 slices bread, cut into ½-in. cubes

1. Preheat oven to 300°F. Heat oil and garlic in a large skillet just until garlic starts to sizzle. Remove from heat and add bread cubes. Stir until all oil has been absorbed by the bread. Place the bread in a flat baking pan, and bake in preheated oven for about 25 minutes or until a golden brown, stirring several times for even browning. (Makes 2 cups.)

SERVES 8 (¼-cup servings)

Per Serving:
Calories: 64
% Calories from Fat: 54
Fat (gm): 3.8
Saturated Fat (gm): 0.6
Cholesterol (mg): 0
Sodium (mg): 68
Protein (gm): 1.1
Carbohydrate (gm): 6.3

Exchanges:
Milk: 0.0
Vegetable: 0.0
Fruit: 0.0
Bread: 0.5
Meat: 0.0
Fat: 0.5

Breadcrumbs

This method is for fresh, soft breadcrumbs, which I prefer using for most recipes. To dry bread for dried breadcrumbs, leave the pieces out on a counter for several hours, turning them occasionally. For toasted breadcrumbs, toast the bread or use croutons.

2 slices bread, broken into pieces

1. Put bread into a food processor or blender and process until desired consistency. (Makes 1 cup.)

SERVES 8 (2-tablespoon servings)

Per Serving:
Calories: 17
% Calories from Fat: 12
Fat (gm): 0.2
Saturated Fat (gm): 0.1
Cholesterol (mg): 0
Sodium (mg): 34
Protein (gm): 0.5
Carbohydrate (gm): 3.1

Exchanges:
Milk: 0.0
Vegetable: 0.0
Fruit: 0.0
Bread: 0.25
Meat: 0.0
Fat: 0.0

Rye and Raisin Cereal

This is my favorite hot cereal. I always keep some of it in the freezer in zip-lock baggies, one serving per bag. Then in the morning I just pop a baggie in the microwave for one minute, and I have a truly satisfying breakfast. I like it with a dollop of low-fat ricotta cheese on top, which I included as an optional ingredient.

1½ cups dry rye berries
1 tablespoon ground cinnamon
1½ teaspoons caraway seeds
1 tablespoon vanilla extract
4½ cups water
¾ cup raisins
Low-fat ricotta cheese (optional)

1. Combine all ingredients, except raisins, in a heavy saucepan and bring to a boil over medium heat. Reduce heat to low and cook, covered, 45 minutes, stirring occasionally, and adding a little more water if necessary. Add raisins and continue cooking, covered, 15 more minutes. Serve warm with a dollop of ricotta cheese on top, if desired. (Makes 4 cups.)

SERVES 8 (½-cup servings)

Per Serving:	*Exchanges:*
Calories: 156	Milk: 0.0
% Calories from Fat: 5	Vegetable: 0.0
Fat (gm): 0.9	Fruit: 1.0
Saturated Fat (gm): 0.1	Bread: 1.5
Cholesterol (mg): 0	Meat: 0.0
Sodium (mg): 4	Fat: 0.0
Protein (gm): 5.2	
Carbohydrate (gm): 34.3	

Herbed Quinoa

Quinoa (pronounced keen-wah) is a tiny, bead-shaped, ivory-colored grain with a bland flavor and a slightly chewy texture. It can be used like rice and cooks in half the time. It was the staple of the Incas, who called it "the mother grain." It is hailed by many as "the super grain of the future" because it contains more protein and is higher in unsaturated fats than most other grains and is a balanced source of many vital nutrients. Quinoa is also considered a complete protein because it contains all eight essential amino acids. This ancient, South American grain is becoming increasingly popular in this country and is available in most supermarkets and all health food stores.

1 14½-ounce can fat-free, sodium-reduced chicken stock

3 tablespoons water

¼ teaspoon freshly ground black pepper

1 cup quinoa

1 tablespoon extra-virgin olive oil

½ teaspoon dried oregano, crushed

¾ teaspoon dried thyme, crushed

1. Combine stock, water, and pepper in a saucepan and bring to a boil. Stir in quinoa, reduce heat to low, and cook, covered, about 12 minutes or until all liquid has been absorbed. Remove from heat and stir in olive oil, oregano, and thyme. Cover again and allow to stand 5 more minutes before serving. (Makes 3 cups.)

SERVES 6 (½-cup servings)

Per Serving:	*Exchanges:*
Calories: 134	Milk: 0.0
% Calories from Fat: 28	Vegetable: 0.0
Fat (gm): 4.3	Fruit: 0.0
Saturated Fat (gm): 0.5	Bread: 1.5
Cholesterol (mg): 0	Meat: 0.0
Sodium (mg): 107	Fat: 0.5
Protein (gm): 5.2	
Carbohydrate (gm): 20.1	

Fast Focaccia

This is a wonderful, homemade "pizza bread" that will take you less than twenty minutes to make.

1 10½-ounce package unbaked pizza dough
1 tablespoon extra-virgin olive oil
¼ cup shredded Parmesan cheese

1. Preheat oven to 400°F. Unroll dough onto a baking sheet, stretching it to fit over entire surface. Push your fingertips lightly into the dough, creating depressions all over the surface. Place dough in preheated oven for 7 minutes.

2. Remove dough from the oven, brush the top with olive oil, and sprinkle cheese evenly over the surface. Place dough back in the oven for about 6 more minutes or until cheese is melted and starting to brown lightly. Remove from oven and cut or break into 12 pieces.

SERVES 12

Per Serving:
Calories: 82
% Calories from Fat: 28
Fat (gm): 2.5
Saturated Fat (gm): 0.5
Cholesterol (mg): 1.6
Sodium (mg): 158
Protein (gm): 3
Carbohydrate (gm): 11.3

Exchanges:
Milk: 0.0
Vegetable: 0.0
Fruit: 0.0
Bread: 1.0
Meat: 0.0
Fat: 0.5

Make-Ahead Florida French Toast

This is a terrific breakfast to prepare for house guests because you can make it the night before and put a sensational meal on the table in just minutes.

12 slices French bread (¾" thick)

1 cup non-fat liquid egg substitute

1 12-ounce can evaporated skim milk

1 tablespoon sugar

¼ teaspoon canola oil

¼ cup orange juice

1 teaspoon grated orange rind

1 teaspoon vanilla extract

Powdered sugar, to taste

1. Place bread slices in a 9 x 13-in. baking dish. In a medium bowl, combine all remaining ingredients, except powdered sugar, and beat until well mixed. Pour over bread, turning slices to coat evenly. Cover and refrigerate overnight.

2. Spray a large, non-stick skillet with non-stick vegetable cooking spray. Place skillet over medium-low heat until water dances on the surface. Cook soaked bread slices about 3 at a time, so as not to crowd skillet, until bread turns golden brown on both sides. To serve, sprinkle each slice with powdered sugar, if desired.

SERVES 12 (1-slice servings)

Per Serving:	*Exchanges:*
Calories: 108	Milk: 0.0
% Calories from Fat: 8	Vegetable: 0.0
Fat (gm): 1	Fruit: 0.0
Saturated Fat (gm): 0.2	Bread: 1.0
Cholesterol (mg): 0.9	Meat: 0.5
Sodium (mg): 212	Fat: 0.0
Protein (gm): 6.1	
Carbohydrate (gm): 18.3	

Sourdough Milk Toast with Honeyed Peaches

This dish is truly tasty and proves that you don't have to use eggs to make great "French" toast. Although this recipe calls for peaches, you can use any fresh, canned, or frozen fruit you happen to have on hand. In fact, it is an excellent way to use up over-ripe fruit.

½ cup non-fat dry milk powder

½ cup water

½ teaspoon ground cinnamon

Dash salt

½ teaspoon vanilla extract

4 slices sourdough bread

1 16-ounce can sliced peaches in water, drained

1 tablespoon honey

Ground cinnamon, for garnish

1. Combine milk powder and water and stir until completely dissolved. Stir in cinnamon, salt, and vanilla.

2. Place the bread in a flat dish large enough so that slices do not overlap. Pour milk mixture over the bread and allow to stand 5 minutes. Turn the bread over and allow to soak until most liquid has been absorbed.

3. Spray a large non-stick skillet with non-stick vegetable cooking spray and place it over medium-low heat. When pan is hot enough for drops of water to dance on the surface, carefully place soaked bread slices in it. Pour any remaining liquid over bread. Cook until bottom of bread is nicely browned. Turn over and brown the other side. Remove bread from the skillet and place it on a serving plate.

4. Add peaches and honey to the hot skillet and cook, stirring frequently, 4 minutes. Spoon ¼ of the peaches over each slice of toast and then sprinkle tops lightly with ground cinnamon, if desired. Serve immediately.

SERVES 4 (1-slice servings)

Per Serving:
Calories: 146
% Calories from Fat: 6
Fat (gm): 0.9
Saturated Fat (gm): 0.2
Cholesterol (mg): 1.6
Sodium (mg): 202
Protein (gm): 5.7
Carbohydrate (gm): 29

Exchanges:
Milk: 0.5
Vegetable: 0.0
Fruit: 0.5
Bread: 1.0
Meat: 0.0
Fat: 0.0

Oatmeal Pancakes

These pancakes are as delicious as they are unusual. I always make more than I need and freeze the rest in individual plastic bags. I reheat the frozen pancakes in the toaster when I'm really in a hurry!

1½ cups uncooked, old-fashioned rolled oats

¼ teaspoon salt

½ teaspoon baking powder

½ teaspoon baking soda

1 tablespoon sugar

1 tablespoon ground cinnamon

3 egg whites

1 12-ounce can evaporated skim milk

1 teaspoon vanilla extract

1. In a blender or food processor, process oatmeal to the consistency of coarse flour. Put oat "flour" in a large bowl. Add all other dry ingredients and mix well.

2. In another bowl, combine egg whites, milk, and vanilla and mix well. Pour liquid ingredients into dry ingredients and stir until completely moistened.

3. Heat a large non-stick skillet or griddle over medium-low heat until drops of water dance on surface. Spoon on 3 tablespoons of batter for each pancake, and cook until golden brown on both sides.

SERVES 6 (2-pancake servings)

Per Serving:
Calories: 142
% Calories from Fat: 18
Fat (gm): 1.4
Saturated Fat (gm): 0.2
Cholesterol (mg): 1.8
Sodium (mg): 316
Protein (gm): 9.4
Carbohydrate (gm): 22.8

Exchanges:
Milk: 0.0
Vegetable: 0.0
Fruit: 0.0
Bread: 2.0
Meat: 0.0
Fat: 0.0

Breakfast Pizza

Children love this quick and easy treat for after-school snacks as well as for breakfast.

1 whole wheat English muffin
¼ cup no-sugar-added, all-fruit jam
½ cup grated low-fat mozzarella cheese

1. Cut muffin in half and roll it out with a rolling pin until much flatter and larger in diameter. Toast muffin, cut side up, under broiler. Spread 2 tablespoons of jam on each toasted muffin half. Sprinkle ¼ cup of grated cheese on top of jam. Place muffin halves back under the broiler until cheese is melted and very lightly browned. Serve immediately.

SERVES 2

Per Serving:
Calories: 236
% Calories from Fat: 14
Fat (gm): 3.7
Saturated Fat (gm): 0.1
Cholesterol (mg): 10
Sodium (mg): 365
Protein (gm): 11.1
Carbohydrate (gm): 42.4

Exchanges:
Milk: 0.0
Vegetable: 0.0
Fruit: 1.5
Bread: 1.0
Meat: 1.0
Fat: 0.0

Southern Bacon Cornbread

This cornbread can be made like a snackin' cake. Line the pan with foil, allowing at least six inches to overhang on all four sides. When the cornbread is cool, wrap it up in the foil for a perfect portable snack for picnics and tailgate parties.

1 cup yellow cornmeal

1 cup unbleached, all-purpose flour

½ teaspoon salt

¼ teaspoon freshly ground black pepper

1 tablespoon baking powder

¼ cup imitation bacon chips

1 cup non-fat milk

1 egg

2 tablespoons canola, *or* corn, oil

3 tablespoons honey

1 cup frozen corn, *or* 1, 8¾-ounce can salt-free corn, drained

1. Preheat oven to 375°F. Spray an 8 x 8-in. (or 7 x 11-in.) pan with non-stick vegetable cooking spray and set aside. Combine cornmeal, flour, salt, pepper, baking powder, and bacon chips in a bowl and mix well.

2. In another bowl, combine all remaining ingredients, mix well, and add to dry ingredients. Stir until thoroughly moistened; do not over mix. Spoon mixture into the prepared pan and bake in preheated oven 25 minutes or until golden brown. Cool on a rack at least 10 minutes before turning out onto a cutting board and cutting into 8 pieces.

SERVES 8

Per Serving:	*Exchanges:*
Calories: 218	Milk: 0.0
% Calories from Fat: 22	Vegetable: 0.0
Fat (gm): 5.6	Fruit: 0.0
Saturated Fat (gm): 0.7	Bread: 2.5
Cholesterol (mg): 27.1	Meat: 0.0
Sodium (mg): 370	Fat: 1.0
Protein (gm): 6.2	
Carbohydrate (gm): 37.1	

NINE

Snacks, Sweets,

AND

Desserts

*This is a small collection of truly tasty and satisfying desserts that
can all be made spur of the moment with ingredients from either your
dry pantry, refrigerator, or freezer. You may find that some of them will
become part of your everyday repertory no matter how
much time you have to make dessert.*

Secret Sauce ◎ Orange Meringue Sauce ◎ Whipped Maple
Topping ◎ Low-Fat Chocolate Sauce ◎ Fiesta Grapefruit Tropical
Fruit Compote ◎ Prune Pudding ◎ Peach Risotto
Italian Cheesecake ◎ Strawberry-Rhubarb Crisp
Unbaked Peach Pie ◎ Piña Colada Pie ◎ Crustless
Shoofly Pie ◎ Frozen Peanut Butter Pie ◎ Lacy
Oatmeal Cookies ◎ Granola-Peanut Candy

Secret Sauce

This sauce is my own "secret weapon." Whenever I don't have anything for dessert, I just open a can of fruit and spoon some Secret Sauce over the top. Guests always think it is an outrageously rich crème anglaise. *You can vary the flavor of the sauce according to what you are using it on. For example, you may want to use the Grand Marnier called for in this recipe for berries, Amaretto for peaches, and a little brandy for prunes.*

    1 cup melted vanilla ice milk

    1½ teaspoons Grand Marnier, *or* any orange-flavored liqueur

1. Combine melted ice milk and liqueur and mix well. (Makes 1 cup.)

SERVES 8 (2-tablespoon servings)

Per Serving:	*Exchanges:*
Calories: 39	Milk: 0.0
% Calories from Fat: 17	Vegetable: 0.0
Fat (gm): 0.7	Fruit: 0.0
Saturated Fat (gm): 0.5	Bread: 0.5
Cholesterol (mg): 3.2	Meat: 0.0
Sodium (mg): 20	Fat: 0.0
Protein (gm): 1.4	
Carbohydrate (gm): 6.5	

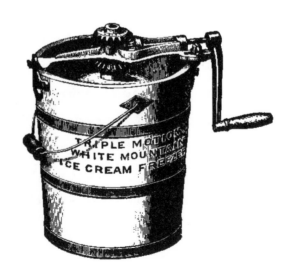

Orange Meringue Sauce

This fabulous, satin-smooth meringue can be used as a sauce or a dip for fruit or cake, or served like a sherbet. For a really incredible dessert, try topping it with drained mandarin orange segments and a little Secret Sauce flavored with Grand Marnier. This meringue is made with Just Whites, a shelf-stable dry powdered egg white. It is a completely natural product made only from egg whites and contains no additives or preservatives. It is also salmonella-negative because it is pasteurized and therefore can be used in recipes calling for uncooked raw egg whites.

¾ cup frozen orange juice concentrate, undiluted, slightly warmed

¼ cup egg white powder

½ cup sugar

1. Combine warmed orange juice concentrate and egg white powder and mix well. Using an electric beater, beat mixture until it starts to thicken. Slowly add sugar and continue beating until soft peaks form. (Makes about 2 cups.)

SERVES 8 (¼-cup servings)

Per Serving:
Calories: 104
% Calories from Fat: 0
Fat (gm): 0.1
Saturated Fat (gm): 0
Cholesterol (mg): 0
Sodium (mg): 48
Protein (gm): 3.3
Carbohydrate (gm): 22.8

Exchanges:
Milk: 0.0
Vegetable: 0.0
Fruit: 1.5
Bread: 0.0
Meat: 0.5
Fat: 0.0

Whipped Maple Topping

You can alter the flavor of this versatile dessert topping by replacing the maple syrup with either sugar or honey. It is also a tasty topping for pancakes and waffles.

1 10½-ounce package silken-firm tofu

3 tablespoons maple syrup

1 teaspoon vanilla extract

⅛ teaspoon ground cinnamon

1. Combine all ingredients in a blender and blend satin smooth. Cover and refrigerate at least 30 minutes before using unless you're putting it on something hot. (Makes 1½ cups.)

SERVES 12 (2-tablespoon servings)

Per Serving:	*Exchanges:*
Calories: 28	Milk: 0.0
% Calories from Fat: 21	Vegetable: 0.0
Fat (gm): 0.7	Fruit: 0.0
Saturated Fat (gm): 0.1	Bread: 0.5
Cholesterol (mg): 0	Meat: 0.0
Sodium (mg): 9	Fat: 0.0
Protein (gm): 1.7	
Carbohydrate (gm): 3.9	

Low-Fat Chocolate Sauce

This sauce thickens when chilled and is wonderful served over ice milk, frozen yogurt, or sliced angel food cake—use your imagination!

½ cup cocoa

½ cup sugar

½ cup corn syrup

½ cup non-fat milk

½ teaspoon vanilla extract

1. Combine all ingredients, except vanilla extract, in a saucepan and bring to a boil over medium-low heat. Remove from heat and stir in vanilla. Cover and refrigerate until cold. (Makes 1⅓ cups.)

SERVES 10 (2-tablespoon servings)

Per Serving:
Calories: 100
% Calories from Fat: 4
Fat (gm): 0.4
Saturated Fat (gm): 0.1
Cholesterol (mg): 0.2
Sodium (mg): 21
Protein (gm): 1.2
Carbohydrate (gm): 25.1

Exchanges:
Milk: 0.0
Vegetable: 0.0
Fruit: 0.0
Bread: 1.5
Meat: 0.0
Fat: 0.0

Fiesta Grapefruit

This is a delightfully refreshing dessert. It is particularly good following a Mexican or Southwestern meal.

    1 16-ounce can grapefruit sections, packed in juice
    1 tablespoon Kaluha
    Whole coffee beans for garnish (optional)

1. Drain grapefruit sections, reserving 1 tablespoon of the juice from can. Combine drained grapefruit, the tablespoon of juice, and Kaluha in a bowl and mix well. Cover and refrigerate until cold. (Makes 1⅓ cups.)

SERVES 4 (⅓-cup servings)

Per Serving:
Calories: 57
% Calories from Fat: 2
Fat (gm): 0.1
Saturated Fat (gm): 0
Cholesterol (mg): 0
Sodium (mg): 9
Protein (gm): 0.8
Carbohydrate (gm): 12.5

Exchanges:
Milk: 0.0
Vegetable: 0.0
Fruit: 1.0
Bread: 0.0
Meat: 0.0
Fat: 0.0

Tropical Fruit Compote

At first glance this may not look like a real pantry recipe because of the banana. However, I always keep sealed bags of sliced bananas in my freezer to make the Banana Shake in the beverage section, and they work beautifully for this recipe, too.

1 cup plain, non-fat yogurt
1 banana, peeled, sliced
1 20-ounce can pineapple chunks, packed in juice, chilled and drained
Ground cinnamon, for garnish (optional)

1. Combine yogurt and banana in a blender or food processor and blend until smooth. Pour mixture over drained pineapple chunks and sprinkle a little cinnamon over top of each serving, if desired. (Makes 2 cups.)

SERVES 4 (½-cup servings)

Per Serving:	*Exchanges:*
Calories: 143	Milk: 0.5
% Calories from Fat: 2	Vegetable: 0.0
Fat (gm): 0.4	Fruit: 1.5
Saturated Fat (gm): 0.1	Bread: 0.0
Cholesterol (mg): 1	Meat: 0.0
Sodium (mg): 46	Fat: 0.0
Protein (gm): 4.1	
Carbohydrate (gm): 33.3	

Prune Pudding

This is a really rich-tasting dish that can be made to taste even richer by pouring a little Secret Sauce (see page 138) flavored with brandy over each serving.

1 cup pitted prunes (about 18)

¾ cup boiling water

1 envelope unflavored gelatin

2 tablespoons cool water

¼ cup boiling water

¾ cup non-fat, dry milk powder

1 cup water

½ teaspoon ground cinnamon

1 teaspoon vanilla extract

1. Combine prunes and ¾ cup boiling water in a bowl. Cover and allow to stand at least 1 hour.

2. Soften gelatin in 2 tablespoons of cool water. Add ¼ cup boiling water and stir until gelatin is completely dissolved.

3. Put prunes and all of the liquid in the bowl of a blender or food processor. Add dissolved gelatin and all remaining ingredients and blend until satin smooth. Pour mixture into a bowl or individual cups or molds, and refrigerate at least 3 hours before serving. (Makes 3 cups.)

SERVES 6 (½-cup servings)

Per Serving:
Calories: 102
% Calories from Fat: 2
Fat (gm): 0.2
Saturated Fat (gm): 0.1
Cholesterol (mg): 1.6
Sodium (mg): 49
Protein (gm): 4.7
Carbohydrate (gm): 21.7

Exchanges:
Milk: 0.5
Vegetable: 0.0
Fruit: 1.0
Bread: 0.0
Meat: 0.0
Fat: 0.0

Peach Risotto

Risotto works just as well in the sweet range as it does in the savory range—this delicious and unusual dessert being a great example.

> 1 8-ounce can sliced peaches packed in water, no sugar added, undrained
> 1 tablespoon corn oil margarine
> ½ cup uncooked arborio rice
> 2 tablespoons dark rum
> ¾ cup apple juice
> 1 tablespoon dark brown sugar
> ¼ teaspoon ground cinnamon
> ⅛ teaspoon salt
> 1 12-ounce can evaporated skim milk, warmed
> 1 teaspoon vanilla extract

1. Drain peaches, reserving liquid. Dice drained peaches and set aside to add later.

2. Melt margarine in a heavy saucepan over medium heat. Add rice and stir 1 minute to coat each grain with margarine. Add rum and cook, stirring constantly, until almost dry. Continuing to stir, add reserved liquid from peaches and again cook until almost dry. Then add ½ of apple juice and reduce until almost dry. Add remaining apple juice, diced peaches, brown sugar, cinnamon, and salt and again reduce until most of the liquid is gone.

3. Start adding warm milk, ½ cup at a time, always stirring frequently, until most of the milk has been absorbed before adding more. There should always be a veil of liquid over the top. This process will take about 20 minutes.

4. Do not allow the last addition of milk to be completely absorbed. Risotto should have a creamy, cereal-like consistency. Remove from heat and stir in the vanilla. Serve warm as a real risotto or refrigerate and serve cold as a creamy rice pudding. (Makes 2 cups.)

SERVES 4 (½-cup servings)

Per Serving:		Exchanges:	
Calories: 248		Milk: 0.5	
% Calories from Fat: 12		Vegetable: 0.0	
Fat (gm): 3.2		Fruit: 1.0	
Saturated Fat (gm): 0.6		Bread: 1.5	
Cholesterol (mg): 2.7		Meat: 0.0	
Sodium (mg): 203		Fat: 0.5	
Protein (gm): 8.3			
Carbohydrate (gm): 41.7			

Italian Cheesecake

I also call this recipe "Short Cut" Cheesecake because it is so easy to make.

1 30-ounce container non-fat ricotta cheese

1¼ cups liquid egg substitute (divided)

¾ cup sugar

1 20-ounce box lemon cake mix

1⅓ cups water

3 tablespoons powdered sugar

1. Preheat oven to 350°F. Spray a 9 x 13-in. baking dish with non-stick vegetable cooking spray.

2. In a large bowl, beat together ricotta cheese, ¾ cup of the egg substitute, and sugar. Set aside.

3. In another large mixing bowl, combine cake mix, water, and remaining ½ cup egg substitute. Using an electric mixer, beat at low speed until moistened, about 30 seconds. Beat at medium speed for 2 more minutes. Pour mixture into the prepared baking dish. Spoon cheese mixture evenly over the top of the batter.

4. Bake in preheated oven 60 to 65 minutes or until the edges are lightly browned and the center is only slightly wiggly. Cool on a rack until room temperature, and then refrigerate several hours before cutting. To serve, put powdered sugar in a strainer and sprinkle evenly over top.

SERVES 15

Per Serving:
Calories: 252
% Calories from Fat: 13
Fat (gm): 3.8
Saturated Fat (gm): 0
Cholesterol (mg): 6.1
Sodium (mg): 289
Protein (gm): 11.3
Carbohydrate (gm): 44.6

Exchanges:
Milk: 0.0
Vegetable: 0.0
Fruit: 0.0
Bread: 3.0
Meat: 1.0
Fat: 0.0

Strawberry-Rhubarb Crisp

This rich-tasting, old-fashioned dessert is best served warm. I like to top it with a dollop of either a non-dairy whipped topping or non-fat frozen yogurt.

Filling

    1 16-ounce package frozen unsweetened strawberries, thawed
    1 16-ounce package frozen unsweetened rhubarb, thawed
    ⅔ cup sugar
    ¼ cup minute tapioca
    ½ teaspoon ground cinnamon
    ¼ teaspoon ground ginger
    2 teaspoons vanilla extract

Topping

    ⅔ cup rolled oats
    ⅔ cup whole wheat flour
    ⅔ cup light brown sugar
    ½ teaspoon ground cinnamon
    ¼ teaspoon ground ginger
    ⅛ teaspoon salt
    3 tablespoons cold corn oil margarine

1. Preheat oven to 375°F. Spray an 8 x 8-in. baking pan with non-stick vegetable cooking spray.

2. Combine strawberries, rhubarb, sugar, tapioca, cinnamon, ginger, and vanilla in large bowl and mix well. Spoon mixture into prepared pan.

3. In another bowl, combine all topping ingredients, except margarine, and mix well. Add margarine and mix, using a pastry blender or fork, until the consistency of gravel. Spoon mixture over ingredients in the pan and bake in preheated oven about 50 minutes or until golden brown. Serve warm or at room temperature. Store covered in refrigerator.

SERVES 9 (½-cup servings)

Per Serving:	*Exchanges:*
Calories: 252	Milk: 0.0
% Calories from Fat: 16	Vegetable: 0.0
Fat (gm): 4.5	Fruit: 1.0
Saturated Fat (gm): 0.7	Bread: 2.0
Cholesterol (mg): 0	Meat: 0.0
Sodium (mg): 84	Fat: 1.0
Protein (gm): 2.9	
Carbohydrate (gm): 52.4	

Unbaked Peach Pie

This quick and easy-to-make pie is amazingly rich tasting considering how low in fat it is.

½ cup graham cracker crumbs

1 envelope unflavored gelatin

2 tablespoons cool water

¼ cup boiling water

¾ cup low-fat cottage cheese

3 tablespoons light brown sugar

¼ teaspoon ground cinnamon

1 teaspoon vanilla extract

½ teaspoon almond extract

1 16-ounce bag frozen peaches, thawed

2 teaspoons ground cinnamon

1. Preheat oven to 350°F. Spray a 9-in. pie plate with non-stick vegetable cooking spray. Add graham cracker crumbs, tilting the plate to cover entire inner surface. Bake in preheated oven about 7 minutes or until nicely browned. Cool on a rack.

2. Soften gelatin in cool water 5 minutes. Add boiling water and stir until completely dissolved. Combine dissolved gelatin and all remaining ingredients, except peaches, in a blender and blend until smooth. Add ½ cup peaches to the blender and again blend until smooth. Transfer to a bowl and stir in remaining peaches.

3. Pour mixture into the cooled pie plate. Sprinkle top lightly with cinnamon and refrigerate until firm before serving.

SERVES 8

Per Serving:
Calories: 99
% Calories from Fat: 10
Fat (gm): 1.2
Saturated Fat (gm): 0.1
Cholesterol (mg): 0.9
Sodium (mg): 129
Protein (gm): 4.3
Carbohydrate (gm): 18.3

Exchanges:
Milk: 0.0
Vegetable: 0.0
Fruit: 0.5
Bread: 1.0
Meat: 0.0
Fat: 0.0

Piña Colada Pie

This easy-to-make pie is so delicious that it is sure to be a big hit after any meal. However, it is particularly good with Asian- or Caribbean-inspired menus.

1 envelope unflavored gelatin

2 tablespoons cool water

¼ cup boiling water

3 tablespoons non-fat, dry milk powder

¼ cup cool water

½ cup fat-free cottage cheese

1 teaspoon vanilla extract

1 teaspoon coconut extract

1 tablespoon sugar

1 20-ounce can crushed pineapple in juice, drained

1 baked graham cracker crust, purchased

2 teaspoons ground cinnamon

1. Soften gelatin in 2 tablespoons of cool water. Add ¼ cup boiling water and stir until completely dissolved. Combine all remaining ingredients, except pie crust and cinnamon, in a blender and blend until smooth. Pour mixture into the pie crust and sprinkle top with cinnamon. Refrigerate at least 3 hours before serving.

SERVES 8

Per Serving:
Calories: 184
% Calories from Fat: 27
Fat (gm): 5.7
Saturated Fat (gm): 1.1
Cholesterol (mg): 0.9
Sodium (mg): 195
Protein (gm): 4.6
Carbohydrate (gm): 29.3

Exchanges:
Milk: 0.0
Vegetable: 0.0
Fruit: 1.0
Bread: 1.0
Meat: 0.0
Fat: 1.0

Crustless Shoofly Pie

This very inexpensive and easy-to-make Southern dessert supposedly got its name because it was so sweet that it was hard to keep the flies away. It is usually made in a very rich pastry shell, which, of course, adds enormously to the total fat content of the pie and *it takes more time to make! I suggest placing the pie plate on a baking sheet because the pie occasionally boils over, and it's a great deal easier to clean the baking sheet than the oven!*

¾ cup boiling water

1½ teaspoons baking soda

½ cup dark corn syrup

1 egg white, lightly beaten

¾ cup flour

½ cup dark brown sugar

¼ teaspoon salt

½ teaspoon ground cinnamon

¼ teaspoon ground nutmeg

⅛ teaspoon ground ginger

⅛ teaspoon ground clove

2 tablespoons cold corn oil margarine

1. Preheat oven to 400°F. Spray a 10-in. pie pan with non-stick vegetable cooking spray and set aside.

2. Combine boiling water and baking soda and stir until completely dissolved. Add dark corn syrup and egg white and mix well.

3. In another bowl, combine all remaining ingredients and mix, using a pastry blender or fork, until the consistency of coarse meal. Place alternate layers of liquid mixture and dry mixture in the prepared pan, ending with the dry mixture as the top layer.

4. Bake on a baking sheet in the preheated oven 20 minutes. Reduce heat to 300°F. and continue baking 20 more minutes or until firm. Cool on a wire rack until room temperature. Store covered in refrigerator.

SERVES 8

Per Serving:	*Exchanges:*
Calories: 184	Milk: 0.0
% Calories from Fat: 15	Vegetable: 0.0
Fat (gm): 3	Fruit: 0.0
Saturated Fat (gm): 0.5	Bread: 2.0
Cholesterol (mg): 0	Meat: 0.0
Sodium (mg): 189	Fat: 0.5
Protein (gm): 1.7	
Carbohydrate (gm): 37.7	

Frozen Peanut Butter Pie

This is a lighter version of a recipe given to me by the wife of a Georgia peanut farmer when I was a guest for dinner in their home. It is a quick, easy, and sinfully delicious dessert that you can keep in the freezer for unexpected guests or for those occasions when you just don't have time to make dessert for your family. However, plan to serve this pie after a very low-fat meal because even though it is much lower in fat than the original recipe, it is still a relatively high-fat dessert.

1 8-ounce carton fat-free cream cheese

½ cup unhomogenized (old-fashioned) smooth peanut butter

⅔ cup confectioner's sugar

2 tablespoons non-fat dry milk powder

¼ cup water

6 ounces (½ of 12-ounce container) low-fat frozen whipped topping, thawed

1 9-in. baked graham cracker crust, purchased

2 tablespoons crushed peanuts, for garnish (optional)

1. Put cream cheese in a large bowl and use an electric mixer to whip it until fluffy. Add peanut butter and sugar and whip until smooth. Dissolve dry milk in the water and slowly whip it into the mixture. Fold in whipped topping until no streaks of white show.

2. Spoon mixture into the crust and top with crushed peanuts, if desired. Cover and freeze all day or overnight. To serve, remove from freezer and allow to soften 15 minutes before cutting.

SERVES 8

Per Serving:	*Exchanges:*
Calories: 328	Milk: 0.0
% Calories from Fat: 45	Vegetable: 0.0
Fat (gm): 16.6	Fruit: 0.0
Saturated Fat (gm): 2.6	Bread: 2.0
Cholesterol (mg): 3.7	Meat: 1.0
Sodium (mg): 445	Fat: 3.0
Protein (gm): 10.8	
Carbohydrate (gm): 35.1	

Lacy Oatmeal Cookies

These delicate-looking cookies are so good they may be habit forming. You can also add chopped nuts and/or raisins if you wish.

1 egg

1 egg white

¾ teaspoon vanilla extract

½ cup sugar

¼ cup dark brown sugar

½ teaspoon salt

½ teaspoon ground cinnamon

1½ teaspoons baking powder

1 tablespoon canola oil

1⅓ cups old-fashioned rolled oats

3 tablespoons whole wheat flour

1. Preheat oven to 350°F. Spray 2 baking sheets with a non-stick vegetable cooking spray.

2. Combine egg, egg white, vanilla, sugar, brown sugar, salt, cinnamon, and baking powder in a bowl and beat with an electric beater until satin smooth and slightly increased in volume. Fold in oil, oats, and flour.

3. Drop by tablespoonfuls onto prepared sheets and bake in preheated oven 10 to 12 minutes or until golden brown. Using a spatula, immediately remove cookies from baking sheets and allow to cool before serving.

SERVES 24 (1-cookie servings)

Per Serving:	Exchanges:
Calories: 55	Milk: 0.0
% Calories from Fat: 17	Vegetable: 0.0
Fat (gm): 1.1	Fruit: 0.0
Saturated Fat (gm): 0.2	Bread: 1.0
Cholesterol (mg): 8.9	Meat: 0.0
Sodium (mg): 71	Fat: 0.5
Protein (gm): 1.3	
Carbohydrate (gm): 10.3	

Granola-Peanut Candy

¼ cup honey

¼ cup unhomogenized peanut butter

¾ cup fat-free granola

1 cup puffed cereal, wheat or rice

1. In a large saucepan, bring honey to a boil. Immediately remove pan from the heat and stir in peanut butter. Add granola and puffed cereal and mix well.

2. Spoon mixture into a standard-size loaf pan, which has been sprayed with non-stick vegetable cooking spray. Moisten your hands and press mixture down to make an even, firm layer.

3. Refrigerate several hours or overnight. Turn out onto a cutting board and cut into 32 squares. If pieces start to crumble, just press them back together again. Store candy in refrigerator.

SERVES 32 (1-piece servings)

Per Serving:	Exchanges:
Calories: 30	Milk: 0.0
% Calories from Fat: 29	Vegetable: 0.0
Fat (gm): 1	Fruit: 0.0
Saturated Fat (gm): 0.2	Bread: 0.5
Cholesterol (mg): 0	Meat: 0.0
Sodium (mg): 12	Fat: 0.0
Protein (gm): 0.8	
Carbohydrate (gm): 4.9	

TEN

Beverages

Whether you're looking for a non-alcoholic cocktail, breakfast in a glass, or fancy pantry coffee—you'll find it in this chapter.

Pilot's Cocktail ⟲ Spiced Cider ⟲ Bloody Mary Mix ⟲ Fruit Frappé ⟲ Banana Shake Peanut Butter Shake ⟲ Honeyed Strawberry Flip Café au Lait

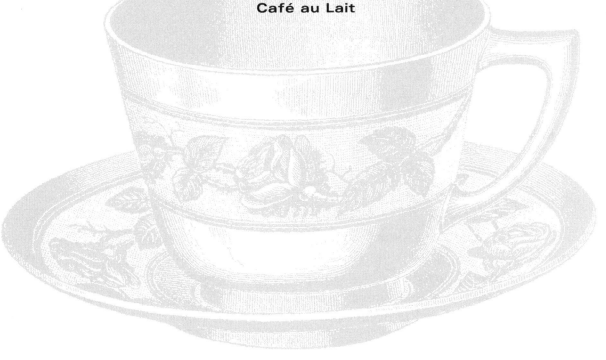

Pilot's Cocktail

This is a refreshing, non-alcoholic beverage that both looks and tastes like a "real" drink. It is aptly named for the person in control of the airplane who cannot drink alcoholic beverages either before or during flight. The Pilot's Cocktail is also perfect for the designated driver on the ground!

    1 cup Perrier, *or* other sparkling water, cold
    Angostura bitters, to taste
    Lime, *or* lemon, juice (optional)

1. Pour cold sparkling water in a glass and add just a few drops of bitters, or to taste. If you wish, add a few drops of lime or lemon juice. (Makes 1 cup.)

SERVES 1

Per Serving:	*Exchanges:*
Calories: 0	Milk: 0.0
% Calories from Fat: 0	Vegetable: 0.0
Fat (gm): 0	Fruit: 0.0
Saturated Fat (gm): 0	Bread: 0.0
Cholesterol (mg): 0	Meat: 0.0
Sodium (mg): 3	Fat: 0.0
Protein (gm): 0	
Carbohydrate (gm): 0	

Spiced Cider

This versatile drink is wonderful served hot on cold winter nights and delightfully refreshing served cold on hot summer afternoons. Try adding a little sparkling water to it when serving it cold for a Sparkling Spiced Cider.

    1 qt. apple cider, *or* apple juice
    10 whole allspice
    10 whole cloves
    2 cinnamon sticks, broken into pieces

1. Combine all ingredients in a saucepan and bring to a boil over medium heat. Reduce to low and simmer, covered, 10 minutes. Serve hot, or cool to room temperature and refrigerate until cold. (Makes 4 cups.)

SERVES 4 (1-cup servings)

Per Serving:
Calories: 127
% Calories from Fat: 2
Fat (gm): 0.4
Saturated Fat (gm): 0.1
Cholesterol (mg): 0
Sodium (mg): 9
Protein (gm): 0.3
Carbohydrate (gm): 35

Exchanges:
Milk: 0.0
Vegetable: 0.0
Fruit: 2.0
Bread: 0.0
Meat: 0.0
Fat: 0.0

Bloody Mary Mix

This spicy beverage gives a snappy start to your day without the vodka.

1 46-ounce can V-8 juice

¾ cup lemon juice

1½ teaspoons Worcestershire sauce

½ teaspoon freshly ground black pepper

¼ cup prepared horseradish

1. Combine all ingredients and mix well. Refrigerate until cold before serving. (Makes 7 cups.)

SERVES 7 (1-cup servings)

Per Serving:
Calories: 48
% Calories from Fat: 0
Fat (gm): 0
Saturated Fat (gm): 0
Cholesterol (mg): 0
Sodium (mg): 733
Protein (gm): 0.3
Carbohydrate (gm): 10.8

Exchanges:
Milk: 0.0
Vegetable: 2.0
Fruit: 0.0
Bread: 0.0
Meat: 0.0
Fat: 0.0

Fruit Frappé

When you're in a hurry in the morning, this is a wonderful, and portable, break-fast in a glass. Choose the fruit you like best.

> 1 12-ounce can evaporated skim milk
>
> 1 8-ounce can fruit packed in water, no sugar added, undrained
>
> 1 teaspoon sugar
>
> ¼ teaspoon vanilla extract
>
> 3 ice cubes, *or* ½ cup crushed ice

1. Combine all ingredients in a blender and blend until ice is completely pulverized and the drink is thick and frothy. (Makes 3 cups.)

SERVES 3 (1-cup servings)

Per Serving:
Calories: 114
% Calories from Fat: 2
Fat (gm): 0.3
Saturated Fat (gm): 0.1
Cholesterol (mg): 3.6
Sodium (mg): 134
Protein (gm): 8.9
Carbohydrate (gm): 19

Exchanges:
Milk: 1.0
Vegetable: 0.0
Fruit: 0.5
Bread: 0.0
Meat: 0.0
Fat: 0.0

Banana Shake

I always keep plastic bags of sliced bananas in my freezer. I put one-half banana (about one-half cup) into each bag, which is the amount I need to make this high-calcium, high-potassium drink. For an even richer, higher-calcium shake, use non-fat milk instead of water in this recipe. This drink is also a sensational topping for dry cereal. In fact, I like it better than the usual combination of sliced bananas and milk on cereal because the banana flavor is more intense.

½ (½ cup) frozen sliced banana

⅔ cup water

½ cup non-fat dry milk powder

1. Combine all ingredients in a blender and blend until smooth. (Makes 1½ cups.)

SERVES 1

Per Serving:	*Exchanges:*
Calories: 175	Milk: 1.5
% Calories from Fat: 3	Vegetable: 0.0
Fat (gm): 0.5	Fruit: 1.0
Saturated Fat (gm): 0.3	Bread: 0.0
Cholesterol (mg): 6.2	Meat: 0.0
Sodium (mg): 187	Fat: 0.0
Protein (gm): 12.5	
Carbohydrate (gm): 31.1	

Peanut Butter Shake

If you like peanut butter, you'll love this drink. It is a satisfying breakfast beverage, a great snack, and can even be served in a bowl as a dessert soup. For a richer tasting drink, use non-fat milk in place of the water.

1 cup water

1½ cups non-fat dry milk powder

¼ cup unhomogenized creamy peanut butter

3 tablespoons sugar

1 teaspoon vanilla extract

2 cups crushed ice

Ground cinnamon, for garnish (optional)

1. Combine all ingredients in a blender and mix until smooth. (Makes 3 cups.)

SERVES 4 (¾-cup servings)

Per Serving:	*Exchanges:*
Calories: 226	Milk: 1.0
% Calories from Fat: 32	Vegetable: 0.0
Fat (gm): 8.3	Fruit: 0.0
Saturated Fat (gm): 1.6	Bread: 1.5
Cholesterol (mg): 4.7	Meat: 0.5
Sodium (mg): 215	Fat: 1.0
Protein (gm): 13.2	
Carbohydrate (gm): 25.7	

Honeyed Strawberry Flip

This delicious drink can also be served as a cold soup or as a fruit sauce. I like it over angel food cake for dessert.

1½ cups frozen strawberries

½ cup water

¼ cup non-fat dry milk powder

2 tablespoons lemon juice

2 tablespoons honey

1. Combine all ingredients in a blender and blend until smooth. Serve immediately. (Makes 2 cups.)

SERVES 2 (1-cup servings)

Per Serving:	*Exchanges:*
Calories: 139	Milk: 0.5
% Calories from Fat: 1	Vegetable: 0.0
Fat (gm): 0.2	Fruit: 1.5
Saturated Fat (gm): 0	Bread: 0.0
Cholesterol (mg): 1.6	Meat: 0.0
Sodium (mg): 50	Fat: 0.0
Protein (gm): 3.5	
Carbohydrate (gm): 33	

Café au Lait

Café au lait, pronounced ka-FAY oh-LAY, is French for "coffee with milk" and it is extremely popular in Europe. It is becoming an increasingly popular way to drink coffee here as well, as more and more coffee houses spring up all over the country. It is usually made with equal amounts of coffee and scalded milk. To retain the richness of this beverage and still make it lighter and lower in fat, you can make it with non-fat or low-fat milk instead of whole milk. However my favorite formula for this high-calcium coffee drink is to use canned evaporated skim milk and vanilla-flavored decaffeinated coffee. This caffeine-free coffee with negligible fat still has a truly rich and satisfying flavor, and it is a delightful drink for breakfast or for coffee breaks any time of the day. Café au lait is also a marvelous substitute for dessert following dinner.

1½ cups strongly brewed vanilla-nut decaffeinated coffee
   (use 2 heaping tablespoons ground coffee per cup of water)
1 12-ounce can evaporated skim milk, heated to boiling point
Ground cinnamon, *or* nutmeg, *or* cinnamon sticks, for garnish
   (optional)

1. Combine coffee and scalded milk. Garnish with ground cinnamon or nutmeg or a cinnamon stick, if desired. (Makes 3 cups.)

SERVES 3 (1-cup servings)

Per Serving:	*Exchanges:*
Calories: 91	Milk: 1.0
% Calories from Fat: 2	Vegetable: 0.0
Fat (gm): 0.2	Fruit: 0.0
Saturated Fat (gm): 0.1	Bread: 0.0
Cholesterol (mg): 3.6	Meat: 0.0
Sodium (mg): 134	Fat: 0.0
Protein (gm): 8.7	
Carbohydrate (gm): 13.3	

INDEX